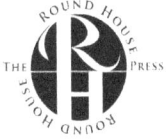

The Round House Press
21 Halls Lane, PO Box 744
Kent, Connecticut 06757
860.927.4390
theroundhousepress@gmail.com
healingcancerbook.com

July, 2009

Dear Friend:

I am delighted to send you the first book to bear the Round House Press imprint. I am not alone in expecting *Healing Cancer Peacefully* to have significant influence as the excesses and incapacities of conventional medicine and the insurance industries come increasingly to light.

Healing Cancer Peacefully is unlikely to be reviewed, at least not fairly, by the Big-Pharma-supported mainstream media. So while we will do our best in that area, I affirm that this book will be lifted into public consciousness largely by enthusiastic word of mouth.

We need the help of our friends for that to happen, so I am asking you to consider writing us a testimonial, a brief blurb to be run in the front pages of the final edition, on the website and on the page where the eBook is offered. This will be enormously valuable.

If you have a friend whose testimonial would be valuable, I ask that you kindly share this copy with him or her, asking that it be passed along for this purpose.

If you will read Dr. Nancy Offenhauser's "Simple, Profound Truths" at the end of Section One, and look at her photo on the back cover, peacefully cancer-free at the age of 60, I believe you will want to do your part to send her revelatory, authoritative light to a very confused and frightened readership.

Healing Cancer Peacefully is, I wholeheartedly believe, today's underline convenient truth. I hope you will agree to lend your name to our inspiring and timely first book.

Many thanks,

Patricia G. Horan
Publisher
The Round House Press

ADVANCE PRAISE FOR
HEALING CANCER PEACEFULLY

"*Healing Cancer Peacefully* is healing the Wise Woman Way, healing by nourishing the wholeness of the unique being, not by waging war against something. Food, story, and ceremony are all needed to nourish and recreate health, as Dr. Offenhauser so clearly shows us. Her story is deep nourishment to each of us and to all of us.

"Buy this book and drink deeply. Green blessings."

> – **Susun S. Weed**, author of *Breast Cancer?*
> *Breast Health! The Wise Woman Way.*

"In her heartful and inspiring story, Nancy Offenhauser shares her deeply personal memoir of healing cancer with us. I was moved, not only by her honesty, but by her courage in trying totally unorthodox treatments as she began to trust her own inner voice over the voices of 'medical authority.' Not only inspiring, *Healing Cancer Peacefully* is also empowering and 'hands on' as it lists the important tools and treatment protocols that Nancy found most useful along the way.

"Most of all, *Healing Cancer Peacefully* is a practical manual that people everywhere can use without fancy equipment or tons of money.

"These are the healing stories we need to hear about cancer— honest, hopeful, and inspiring!"

> – **Rosemary Gladstar**, Herbalist, Founder, United Plant
> Savers, Traditional Medicinals, and Northeast Herbal Assn.,
> Author of *Rosemary Gladstar's Herbal Recipes for Vibrant*
> *Health* and many other books

"This is a very important work. Dr. Nancy Offenhauser must be applauded for her courage, wisdom, and spirit in taking her power regarding her own health in this marvelous book. She beautifully melds her professional analytical knowledge with her emotional human perspective, and has the graceful compassion to share with us all. I hope many people find their way to these pages!"

> – **Pamela Deaver**, M.A., www.flowerempowerment.com

Healing Cancer Peacefully

Healing Cancer Peacefully

When Your Body's Not a Battlefield,
It Can Tell You What It Needs

A Memoir

Nancy Offenhauser, D.C.

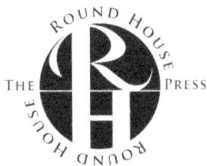

The Round House Press
Kent, Connecticut

Published by
The Round House Press
PO Box 744
Kent, Connecticut 06757

First Edition: June 2009

Offenhauser, Nancy.

Healing cancer peacefully : when your body's not a battlefield, it can tell you what it needs : a memoir / Nancy Offenhauser. -- 1st ed. -- Kent, Conn. : The Round House Press, c2009.

p. ; cm.

ISBN: 978-0-9823089-0-5
Cover title: Healing cancer peacefully : a memoir.
Includes bibliographical references and index.

1. Cancer--Alternative treatment. 2. Cancer--Patients--United States--Biography. 3. Alternative medicine. 4. Mind and body therapies. 5. Herbs--Therapeutic use. I. Title.

RC270.8 .O34 2009   2009922589
616.99/406--dc22   0907

In some cases, names and details have been changed to protect the privacy of the people mentioned in this book.

Design and art direction of covers and Round House Press colophon art direction by Beth Shaw
Interior and cover line illustrations, timeline graph and Round House Press colophon design by Jude Streng
Author photo by Victoria Reap

An eBook Version, ISBN 978-0-9823089-1-2,
is available at www.healingcancerbook.com

www.healingcancerpeacefully.com
www.theroundhousepress.com

Dedication

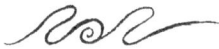

To Sandra and Gwenythe
who showed me it was possible

and

in memory of Doc and L.C.
who taught me how

and

in memory of Bethany Ginsberg Segali
who passes the torch to us

"Any intelligent fool can make things
bigger, more complex, and more violent.
It takes a touch of genius—and a lot of courage—
to move in the opposite direction."
—Albert Einstein

"First, do no harm."
—from the Hippocratic Oath

Table of Contents

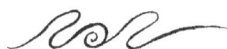

PART I

Viewpoints

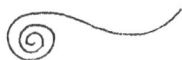

A Disclaimer of Sorts

This book is intended for informational and educational purposes only. It does not replace the services and expertise of a health care professional. It is based on my own experience and research. My experience is my "gold standard," but as soon as it appears in a book it becomes "anecdotal evidence," and the further it strays from the original source, the less reliable it becomes as a standard for anybody else.

I describe a protocol I designed with myself in mind, for my personal and biochemical individuality. Many kinds of cancers exist in a multitude of locations, with a large variation in virulence. The stage at which a cancer is diagnosed is also of vital importance. The farther advanced it is, the more help the body will need to cope with it, and the less energy the patient will have to focus on the work of healing.

There are no guarantees in biology. No two people will respond in the same way to the same intervention. That being said, it is also true that you cannot be wrong in taking steps to improve your general health. Many of the herbs and other interventions I used are not specifically anti-cancer, but instead were used to enhance body function in a number of ways. I am hoping that the Fourteen Points in Section Three and the story that makes up Section Two will provide a new way of thinking about the problem of cancer, from both the preventive and treatment perspectives, and will also provide an opening for discussion with the reader's health care professionals. If so, I will have achieved my goal.

While I never used allopathic medicine in my treatment of cancer, I do not dispute that there are situations in which it is outstanding, particularly in emergencies and in dealing with trauma or severe infection. When surgery is truly indicated, it can be miraculous. Allopathy is far less effective in management of chronic, degenerative disease. My chief objection to allopathic medicine in the treatment of cancer is the arrogance of practitioners who fail to let their patients know about well-established, nonallopathic options, making a joke out of "informed consent," and leading to the perception that the patients have no other choice. Essiac and the Gerson therapy, among others, have been around for more than fifty years.

My second objection to allopathic medicine's treatment of cancer is the failure to look out for the health and vitality of the patient while prescribing toxic, expensive, and destructive "therapies"; this applies to financial as well as physical destruction.

My third objection is the assumption that surgery, radiation, or chemotherapy are always the best choices, and that nutritional, herbal, Chinese medicine, Ayurveda, chiropractic or massage (often totally underrated) therapies should always be "secondary" or "supportive." I eagerly await the day when allopathy learns to collaborate with its elder disciplines and to back off when some other method will provide a neater, cheaper, less stressful, and often far more successful solution to the problem.

One

Invisible Me:
Why I Am Writing This Book

Today is the fifth anniversary of my diagnosis with endometrial cancer. I am officially supposed to be a Cancer Survivor. I think.

I am undoubtedly here, or else I wouldn't be writing this. So I have survived, and in fact am surviving very nicely, thank you. I continue to live normally and work at my chiropractic practice, having been spared mouth sores, hair loss, immune system dysfunction, cachexia—wasting and malnutrition—and all sorts of horrible things. I did have anemia, but reversed it solely by nutritional means, despite continuing to bleed.

However, I doubt you'll see me in statistics anywhere.

Why? There are two simple reasons:

One, I have never been treated by conventional allopathic medicine for this condition. Frankly, I think that's why I'm in such good shape.

Two, the cancer has never been staged. Therefore, in amassing statistics, they can't say I'm a Stage 1A, or a Stage 1B, or a Stage 1C. In order to give me any one of these labels, one of two things has to happen. Either some large piece of tissue has to be removed to be examined by a pathologist, or a CT scan or other toxic test has to be administered to determine the presence or absence of pathology outside the uterus.

I decided not to bother with those options, so you probably won't see me cited in any research study.

Tests need not be invasive

I figured that I knew how rapidly the cancer was progressing (slowly, not at all, or regressing), because I had already been bleeding for over a year at the time of diagnosis and yet still had enough energy to work. So it was not progressing rapidly. My other concern was whether my overall condition was improving or deteriorating. This could be demonstrated simply with two non-toxic and noninvasive tests—AMAS and ultrasound—and by observing my energy level. I didn't need precise information about the size or location of the tumor, because I was not considering surgery. CT scans are often used as a guide for the surgeon to know where to cut.

How many others are out there like me? I suspect there are many. I meet more and more of us. One of my patients is hale and hearty after being given up on by the medical profession thirteen or more years ago "with six months to live," because she didn't believe in surgery. Another refused surgery more than thirty years ago. Both of these women, healthy and not mutilated in any way, confirmed my feeling that the conventional medical approach to treating cancer, consisting of an attempt to heal the body by almost destroying it, is not only counterintuitive, but bordering on insanity. They probably aren't in the statistics either.

Since meeting these two women, I have repeatedly seen, and sometimes been in the position of attempting to remediate, the results of medical treatment of cancer in others. Attempting to remediate the damage done by the treatment, I have discovered, is much more difficult than attempting to remediate the cancer itself.

A particularly dangerous lie

To quote Mark Twain: "There are three kinds of lies: plain lies, damn lies, and statistics."

I'm writing this book to shed light on the particularly dangerous lie that tells us by omission that people don't heal themselves of cancer naturally. I'm writing to shed light on those of us whose survival stories have gone untold. It is of vital importance that the world know about those of us who survive naturally, even peacefully, and even, like me, on a budget.

I discover in my readings that quite a few people have written about their experiences with cancer. Some have used conventional (allopathic) treatments, while others have not. "Allopathy" is defined by *Dorland's Medical Dictionary, 27th Edition,* as "a term applied to that system of therapeutics in which diseases are treated by producing a condition incompatible or antagonistic to the condition to be cured or alleviated. Called also *heteropathy. Cf. homeopathy*" (p.50). In practice, this often seems to consist of using drugs to suppress symptoms, rather than dealing directly with the cause.

The survivors who are of more interest to me have used non-allopathic treatments, and the ones who are of the *most* interest are the ones who have been given up for dead by the allopaths and gone on to lead healthy and happy lives by investigating other means of regaining health.

To begin with, allopathic cancer patients receive a diagnosis of a condition that, according to the definition in *Dorland's Medical Dictionary*, [is] "a cellular tumor, the natural course of which is fatal." (*Dorland's Illustrated Medical Dictionary*, 27th Edition, p.261.) Such patients will usually, therefore, be terrified. Fear induces stress, increasing the production of cortisol, thereby reducing immune function, and a fully functioning immune system is necessary for regaining or maintaining health. So, in such a circumstance, where is hope?

They may also be told that the cause of the cancer is unknown. Where, then, is understanding?

The next message is that the only answer is surgery, chemotherapy or radiation. All of these have to do with tearing down. Chemotherapy, in particular, destroys white blood cells and reduces immune function. Where, then, is building up? If the only answer is surgery, chemotherapy or radiation, where is the control of their lives that people need?

Allopathy, not herbalism, is the new kid on the block

While this Western medical approach to cancer may be conventional and considered orthodox, it is *not* traditional. Chemotherapy and radiation, as practiced today, have been in existence for fewer than one hundred years. Surgery has been around for centuries, and, according to Ralph Moss, Ph.D, in *The Cancer Industry,* "has been practiced since the dawn of history to remove malignancies" (p.43). In many cases, surgery worked but, due to the risks of infection and the brutality of surgery on conscious patients, it only "rose from quackery to respectability in the nineteenth century mainly because of two great discoveries: anesthesia and asepsis" (p.45).

Probably the most truly traditional method of healing cancer is herbalism. Herbs build the body up.

From *Webster's Eleventh Collegiate Dictionary*: "Therapeutic: from the Greek *therapeutikos:* to attend or treat: 1) of or relating to the treatment of disease or disorders by remedial agents or methods; 2) providing or assisting in a cure." I have heard or read many examples of treatment for breast cancer, in particular, in which the initial lumpectomy is followed by chemotherapy and/or radiation. Then, when this doesn't work, the last resort is a bone-marrow transplant. In such a case, chemo or radiation cannot be considered therapies, since they have not worked, and therefore do not meet the definition. So the term "chemotherapy" is itself a lie. This type of treatment is conventional and orthodox (Orthodox: From the Middle English *orthodoxe;* from the Greek *orth-* and *doxa,* opinion: 1a. Conforming to established doctrine, esp. in religion; 1b. Conventional.—*Webster's Eleventh).* However, the fact that it is conventional and orthodox merely means that there has been some sort of consensus declaring it as truth, *not* that it is, in fact, the best or most effective means of solving the problem.

"Treatment" that weakens?

If they are lucky, such allopathic patients may see a doctor who has the time to discuss their life-changing cancer diagnosis compassionately with them. However, in today's insurance- and production-driven culture, there may not be enough time to do this sensitively, and many complain that their doctors don't listen to them. Or do the medical doctors even know how? How frequently are allopathic patients informed of all of their options, allopathic or not?

Once allopathic cancer patients have undergone the conventional medical treatment, they are invariably weakened. Are they then given adequate information to figure out how to rebuild what has been torn down? In many cases, no, though some cancer "treatment" centers are promoting adjunctive "alternative medicine" protocols in an attempt to deal with this issue.

That's fine, as far as it goes, but it doesn't go far enough. Is it really necessary to do all this destruction in the first place? I think not. Why not? Because the emphasis is wrong. I have found, and will demonstrate, that it may not be necessary to kill the cancer, or anything else, in order to get well.

I have had the same basic medical education as any MD, with differences in emphasis. Therefore I can describe and translate test results so that you, if you are a reader without medical education, can understand them. I can talk about the current understanding of various physical and biochemical processes, as I was taught in chiropractic college.

So is *Healing Cancer Peacefully* just one more "how I survived cancer" book? I don't think so. For one thing, I have not only steered clear of conventional medicine, I have also not used anyone's set protocol, alternative or not. Instead I have designed my own, to suit myself. I intend to demonstrate the thought processes I used to do so.

One friend told her doctor that I was treating my cancer by non-medical means. "She's going to die," the doctor said. "And so are you," my friend responded.

Tell me. *How dead do I look to you?*

Two

How I Look at Cancer

Cancer arises out of a state of cell starvation.

Cells require oxygen for their normal metabolic process. Cells turn cancerous after being subjected to a state of hypoxia, or low oxygen, for some time. A low oxygen level can be caused, for example, by poor circulation, lymphatic congestion, or impaired waste removal. These can in turn be created by muscle spasm or disc herniation that causes nerve dysfunction. Infection and toxicity are other potential causes.

Deprived of oxygen, cells switch to the default metabolic pathway, which involves gobbling sugar. This switch to a default mechanism is not unique to cancer cells, by the way. There are other biochemical examples of preferred and secondary pathways being available to achieve a given goal. Usually, however, there is an intrinsic problem with the secondary pathway: It doesn't provide a clean burn. Instead, it creates residues, much like the black smoke that results when logs in a fireplace are burned without enough draft.

Moreover, secondary pathways are intended for emergency use only, and cause long-term problems if used on a permanent basis.

Threatened plants and cells reproduce

Dr. John Donofrio, a chiropractor, told us in our chiropractic board review that "Malignancies eat, reproduce, and don't work." This is consistent behavior for a cell or organism threatened with extinction. Some researchers have reported the social disintegration of indigenous and other groups who have faced starvation. Compassion disappears, with each individual thinking of survival, first and foremost.

Cancer cells, in a state of starvation, behave in a similar fashion. They become greedy. Tumors create their own blood supply, which ultimately takes sustenance away from the rest of the organism. This is a disintegration of the social order within the body. Tumor cells, therefore, "don't work" in their appointed place. They begin to lose the distinctive characteristics of the tissue to which they are supposed to belong, becoming structurally less organized and more chaotic, until they have reverted to an embryonic state, allowing for uncontrolled growth—growth of the group of cells at the expense of the organism as a whole.

Plants threatened by a decrease in the food supply, or simply nearing the end of their growing season, will go to seed in order to reproduce. Cancer cells threatened by starvation will do the same thing.

There's a problem with this. Cancer cells lose track of the distinction between the life of the cell and the life of the organism. A serious error in consciousness has occurred here. The longer the state of starvation continues, the more the cells are going to regress toward the embryonic state. They are renegades, looking out only for themselves. They lose sight of the fact that if the organism dies they will die with it.

Poisoning and burning will not feed or restore order

What will rectify this error in consciousness? Starving, burning, or poisoning them will not encourage the renegade cells to rejoin the social order. It may kill some of them, but if it doesn't kill all of them, the rest will probably respond by either fighting or fleeing to another location where they feel safer. By fleeing to another location, they create metastasis.

The more they feel threatened and are starving, the more the cancer cells are going to gobble. So the logical thing to do is feed them—with oxygen, with real food, with light, with water, with rest, with exercise, with love, with work, with humor, with spiritual practice, with mental endeavor, with meaning.

Little cancers are being formed and hunted down by the immune system all the time. If the individual is in good health, they will be kept under control. However, if low oxygen, poor circulation, poor elimination, nerve interference, infection, or toxicity persist for a long time, the health begins to break down, and the cellular starvation sets in. This creates a cellular panic reaction, which can be exacerbated by the receiving of the diagnosis itself, since people have been conditioned to think that cancer equals death.

Cancer doesn't necessarily equal death. It is, however, a distress call from the body. If you have cancer, it means that something in your life, whether physical or emotional, is intolerable to the body and has to be changed NOW! You have the chance to decide what needs to change and go about changing it. Cancer is a default response. This means that the body will automatically create cancer in an intolerable situation when it doesn't know what else to do. Your body will gladly choose another course, given half a chance, if you are willing to work and negotiate with it. If you do not heed the call to change, the body will begin to travel the path of social disintegration described above.

If your cancer was discovered incidentally on a routine test, chances are it isn't very bad yet. If you consider your cancer as a movie, it makes a huge difference whether you get your diagnosis in the first five minutes, after half an hour, or five minutes from the end. If you are in serious trouble, it may be necessary to use one of the time-tested protocols such as Gerson or Kelley (described below) for rapid and safe detoxification and rebuilding.

Go within and trust your intuition.

Three

If You've Just Been Diagnosed with Cancer

I'd like to talk to you for a minute, before you embark on reading the rest of this book. I recommend that you first...

Take a deep breath.

Realize that fear is a natural response. Also realize that there is much more to the total picture than your doctor is telling you. The Western approach is fear-based, not hope-based, and is only one of many approaches you can take. *Fear depresses your immune system and makes it harder for your body to handle challenges.* So, therefore,

Take another deep breath.

Do nothing. This is the fabulous Step 0 on herbalist and author Susun Weed's decision tree, without which step you cannot make a sound decision. You need time to get yourself accustomed to your new reality. This is the time at which you are most vulnerable to your doctors, family, and friends who might be pressuring you into a course of action that may be best for them, but may not be best for you. Let them state their case. *Once.* Then it may be necessary to withdraw from them and think about things. In most cases, you don't need that expensive and toxic diagnostic test today that may lead up to the expensive, toxic, and invasive course of treatment you may be trapped in tomorrow. You have time to think about it.

Take another deep breath.

Take a good look at where your life is now. What is the cancer telling you that you must change? Think about how you're going to change it.

Now you may be ready to go on to Susun Weed's Step 1: Gather information. A warning here: If what you're reading and hearing in the world at large is too scary, put it aside and go somewhere else. If you're finding Internet chat rooms frightening rather than empowering, avoid them. While you do need a certain amount of medical information about your condition, what you're reading about it may well be a worst-case scenario.

Check out what the herbalists, Chinese herbalists and acupuncturists, naturopaths, chiropractors, alternative medical doctors, and Ayurvedic doctors have to say about it. There is an abundance of material available on alternative methods of treating cancer, with many differing philosophical approaches. Until you have some idea of several of these multiple approaches, along with the conventional Western one, you are NOT prepared to make an informed and balanced decision.

Take another deep breath.

Sit with the information you've gathered for a while. There's a lot of it.

Begin doing things that improve your general physical and mental health. Do what you want. Figure out what that is. Give yourself permission for the long-awaited vacation or change your career to do that thing your heart desires.

Take another deep breath.

Sit with the information a while longer, as you continue to do things that make you feel better. Never underestimate the value of feeling better or the cost of feeling worse.

Listen to your heart. Please only yourself, not anyone else, in making your choices. Don't wait until the eleventh hour before surgery, chemo, etc. to decide whether you really want it. Once you're that far along in that process, it will be increasingly difficult to stop it.

Listen some more to your heart. Pray for and listen to inner guidance.

Take another deep breath.

Continue to gather information. Choose a course that you are free to change if you wish.

Figure out what you need to know, as opposed to what your doctor thinks you need to know, and discuss these differences with him or her. Keep toxic and invasive procedures to a minimum.

Watch movies and read books that make you laugh. Norman Cousins emphasized and popularized this concept. It works.

Others have been on this path before you. Read and listen to as many heartwarming and uplifting success stories as you can.

Remember, you are not alone.

Four

Chiropractic: Drugless Medicine

I am a chiropractor, not an allopath, and in the course of my practice I have become more and more aware of the interconnections of spinal alignment and nervous and visceral function that are central to chiropractic thought. In fourteen years of practice I have discovered that some things I was taught are true, and others are not. I also studied acupuncture for two trimesters, and have used it on patients during my clinical rotation, so while I do not consider myself an acupuncturist, I have some comprehension of the way acupuncture works and how powerful it is.

My style of practice, as it has developed, is not the usual one. While in chiropractic school, I set the intention of listening to each body as closely as I could. This takes time, so I spend about an hour with the average patient. I listen through my hands, which tell me on the simplest physical level about changes in muscle balance. Then, on the next deeper level, they tell me about emotional tone associated with the area on which I am working. Then, on the next deeper level, I may see images or feel feelings from the patient that are associated with the area and have been encoded there. I did the most intense and deepest work of this type with my patient Jean, whose story will be told in these pages, and from whom I learned as much as, or maybe even more than she learned from me.

Most of the time, these stories are from the present lifetime, but occasionally they are from past incarnations. On more than one occasion, the patient and I have alternated telling each other the story, indicating that both of us are seeing the same thing. In much the same way, my late mentor Herbert Spencer ("Doc") Feldman saw auras and colors and predicted cancers two years before diagnosis. Unlike Doc, I do not see auras, but while working on Doc's neck, I could tell when I had improved his circulation because my own vision became brighter. Improving circulation will improve vision. I was seeing through his eyes.

That's how I learn from my patients how their healing processes work, by experiencing them secondhand. From their healing processes, I have learned more about my own.

About chiropractic, and the singular way I work

Chiropractic is a modality that uses adjustment of the spine (a structural intervention) to modulate nervous system function (electrical and chemical). Nervous system function in turn modulates organ function. Chiropractic was founded in the late nineteenth century by D.D. Palmer, who had previously been a magnetic healer and also studied osteopathy with Andrew Taylor Still. Osteopathy was a very new discipline at that time, and chiropractic bears considerable resemblance to it, with some differences in technique and emphasis. At times I may downplay its importance because I take it for granted—when a body part hurts or is malfunctioning, my first response is to adjust it. My second response is to give it the food or supplement I think is most likely to help solve the problem.

I personally do not use pain medication, because it interferes with the communication between the body and the consciousness that is so vital to the healing process. I have taken antibiotics only twice in the last twenty years, once for Lyme disease and once for a dental infection, because I expect that my body can handle most illnesses on its own with the proper rest as well as structural and nutritional support. That is what it is designed to do, and using my own immune system for everyday problems keeps it in tune, making it more likely that I will be able to handle larger ones as well.

If my hand on a patient's neck stimulates a shooting pain down his or her right leg, I get a shooting pain down my right leg, which I then describe to the patient and ask if it's mine or his or hers. If it's not mine, sometimes it relates to an incident in the patient's past and is being used symbolically in some way. I will sometimes get a feeling or see an image, or sometimes I will feel I have to say something. On some occasions, an energetic trace from the patient will persist in my nervous system for twenty-four to forty-eight hours after a treatment, and I will continue to gain insights from this trace until it vanishes. Over time, what can happen is that patients and I figure out the meaning and some of the iconography behind their pain. It all comes down to one thing: Everyone needs to tell his or her story.

Some people see auras. My seeing is through my hands, not my eyes. My hands have taught me about the plasticity of the body, meanings of pain, structure of personality, recording of trauma and, most important, about my patients' individual paths to healing.

I am privileged to be a witness, to be with my patients, to key into their nervous systems, to see what they see, to feel what they feel.

Five

Sing the Magickal Body

The following paragraphs are quite technical in nature. Please bear with me, as I am making a major point here about the built-in changeability of the body. This concept is at the core of my healing journey.

I had my first major religious experience in the Gross Anatomy lab at chiropractic school. We began dissecting cadavers on the second day of class, beginning with the upper thigh. This was good planning for two reasons: one, because the structures there are relatively large and we were less in danger of destroying them due to poor technique. Two, because the rest of the cadaver was draped, and beginning with a part that didn't seem so immediately human made it possible for us to be gradually desensitized, so that, by the end of the second trimester, we were prepared to work on the face and the brain. So, as we separated nerve from muscle, and saw the highly individual pathways taken by the veins, it was possible to focus on the miraculous way in which the body is put together. Up until then I hadn't seen any particular need for the Divine, so didn't pay much attention to it. Then I began to appreciate the brilliance and intricacy of the way the human body is designed. In one way, Gross Anatomy offered very few surprises—I saw over and over again that the design of a body part was perfect for the way in which it needed to function and admired its simplicity and elegance.

Organs tend to be packaged in inner and outer wrappings.

The ear is a better example of miniaturization than any technolgial device human beings have managed to design. The three ossicles—tiny bones, hammer, anvil, and stirrup— in the ear are each the size of a grain of sand. The vibration of these against the eardrum in the middle ear allows for the transfer of sound to the inner ear. Also built in is a mechanism to protect the inner ear from potentially damaging loud sound: The muscles driving the ossicles can be set at varying levels of tension to facilitate or to damp down the vibration. Control of these is usually subconscious, but can also be conscious.

I don't think I could design anything as neatly as that, and I don't know any other human being who could.

So how does healing work?

This is the ultimate mystery. I do not presume to know anything more about it than that. I can, however, offer generally accepted facts and proceed from there to chiropractically accepted findings, personal experiences, stories, extrapolations and conjectures, and in doing so, perhaps shed some light on the subject.

I find that my experience with the healing process over the last thirteen years has shaped my way of coping with cancer, the subject of this book, in many profound ways.

Every day, a miracle

Over the years I've been in practice, I have noticed several key things about the human condition:

First, that physical pain can be the body's way of expressing an emotional issue that needs work, as well as the result of a physical injury.

Second, that physical injury sometimes seems to occur in order that the emotional issue be addressed. I discussed this with a psychotherapist colleague once. He agreed with me that sometimes injury seems to happen to ensure that a deeper, older trauma will be brought to light, worked on, healed. The trauma that is experienced by such an injury may or may not be of the present lifetime. I find it true, and remarkable, that we can have cellular memories deriving from other lifetimes, other bodies. The intelligence directing this is far more profound than our simple, everyday consciousness.

Third, that the depth of healing that can occur is far beyond what one would normally assume could be accomplished by touch and talk.

Fourth, that the problems patients come in with tend to mirror my struggles of the moment more than seems randomly reasonable, and I am changed by my interaction with them.

And fifth, that a patient's condition can be changed by a shift in his or her perception of it.

Describing the healing process doesn't begin to explain it. I can't help believing that something beyond the human is at work here. I see small and not so small miracles every day. I am still in awe any time I feel a healing occurring under my hands. It is still a mystery.

Time and time again, my experience as a chiropractor has shown me evidence of the phenomenal changeability of the body, reinforcing what I had read in the early works of Deepak Chopra, M.D. *(Quantum Healing* is my favorite). As more discoveries are made, it becomes increasingly clear that the human body is much more fluid and changeable than was originally thought.

Bone—even bone!— remodels constantly, according to patterns of use or disuse (which is why weight-bearing exercise is so important for maintaining bone density). Blood cells are made in the marrow. No one knows exactly how living bone operates; it is my experience that it can stretch and twist.

At the beginning of life, bone is mostly cartilage. Ossification isn't complete until about age twenty-five, so young bodies are springy and move easily.

Different tissues in the body slough off and regenerate at different rates. Turnover is rapid in skin, stomach, and hair cells, and growth is also rapid in cancer cells.

Liver cells are capable of regeneration, and it is possible to live with only ten percent of the liver functioning.

Neurotransmitters are found in the gut, as well as in the brain.

Electricity meets chemistry in the body

The body is simultaneously electrical and chemical in nature and runs by an exchange of ions between the cells and the extracellular fluid. Cell membranes are made of fat molecules with polar—hydrophilic—heads and nonpolar—hydrophobic—tails, which can let different things in and out of the cell under different circumstances. Cell membranes are very changeable.

There are two major divisions of the nervous system, the somatic and autonomic. The somatic nervous system is in charge of voluntary motion, while the autonomics modulate organ function. The sympathetic branch of the autonomics handles the "fight or flight" response, while the parasympathetics handle the "relax and repair" response.

The spinal cord, which runs the somatic nervous system, is closely paralleled by the sympathetic nervous system in the thoracics, the vicinity of the twelve vertebrae to which ribs are attached, and lumbars, the five vertebrae of the low back, and the parasympathetic nervous system coming from the cranials and sacrum. Communicating branches run between the somatic and autonomic nervous systems, so they influence each other.

The spinal cord is shock-mounted in the spinal canal. There are three layers of *meninges,* protective coverings for the brain and spinal cord, around it. The outermost, the *dura mater,* lines the canal itself. The middle layer, the *arachnoid*, or spider-like layer, comprises the threads that suspend the cord in the cerebrospinal fluid, and the *pia mater*, which adheres closely to the cord and to the brain.

The spinal cord is bathed in cerebrospinal fluid, which also circulates around the brain. In adults, the spinal cord ends at L1—the first lumbar vertebra— and forms the *cauda equina* (horse's tail), with nerves going out between each of the remaining vertebrae. It begins within the skull, just below the medulla, and is tied off at the coccyx with the *filum terminale,* a part of the *dura mater.*

Muscles support and drive bone. They generally work in opposing pairs, running at a number of angles, allowing a great variety and flexibility of movement. The downside of this is that they are never perfectly balanced.

Muscle tension can influence organ function, and vice versa. Emotional states, in turn, affect muscle tension.

The body's response to anything it doesn't like is universal, regardless of whether the insult is structural, chemical, electrical or emotional: It will always tighten up. The body will reflexively relax, on the other hand, when touched in a non-threatening manner. I use this simple fact in my work all the time.

Even the skull bones move

There are twenty-two bones in the skull. At the beginning of life, these need to be very mobile to allow for some temporary deformation of the skull during the birth process and for the rapid growth that takes place in childhood. The major cranial (as opposed to facial) bones are the frontal, temporal, parietal, and occipital. The frontal and parietal bones are joined by the coronal and midsagittal sutures; the parietal and occipital bones are joined by the lambdoidal suture, and the parietal suture joins the parietal and temporal bones on each side.

I have noticed that, when the cranial bones are very tight, the coronal and midsagittal sutures are often indented. These joints are like interlacing fingers in appearance, similar to expansion joints on bridges, so it appears to me that their function must be to allow motion. In looking at the insides of skulls, I have noticed that there is a ridge under these joints. Does living bone flow? A ridge on the inside could possibly impede the flow of cerebrospinal fluid, so this could be a reason why our brains don't work as well when we are "uptight." I was totally in awe of the design of the skull when we studied it in Neuroanatomy class. A good lecture on the skull is worthy of a round of applause.

The eyes are each suspended by six muscles in their sockets, four rectus and two obliques. Each orbit is made up of seven different bones, so the focus of the eye can change according to the motions of the different bones it's attached to. Three of the twelve cranial nerves are solely devoted to moving these small muscles. I have observed more than once that the focus of the eyes and quality of vision can be adversely affected if the patient has a sinus condition, probably due to pressure from the sinuses moving the bones of the orbit.

Neurons for the sense of smell come directly to the nose from the brain through the cribriform plate, which has holes in it. They can be easily disturbed by an impact to the head and the sense of smell disrupted. The emotional immediacy of smell is a consequence of its direct path to the brain; it is the only sense not routed through the thalamus, the "relay station" between the brain and sensory nerves and between the cerebellum and basal ganglia and the cerebral cortex.

The body takes the hit for the mind

So, if cranial bones move (which they do) and bone remodels according to use or disuse (which it does) and we can direct our circulation at will (which we can) and we can set muscle lengths and tensions either subconsciously or at will, and if we can create new red blood cells to meet additional oxygen demand at higher altitudes (which we can) why should we not be able to use consciousness to affect or reverse a disease process? Consciousness, after all, may well have had a role in creating it.

The body will protect the consciousness from anything the consciousness cannot handle; it does so by burying it in the body. If it is buried, it cannot be healed. The body takes the hit for the consciousness, so that the patient, when discussing the trauma, might say, "It wasn't so bad," whereas the body knows that it was truly awful and is expressing this with severe pain. The first priority, then, is to bring the trauma to consciousness at the proper time. If it's not time yet, the body won't allow it.

The body and the consciousness have different ways of knowing. The body sees only what is very close around it and registers most of its information through feeling, whereas the consciousness sees a wider area around it.

The body will also use an altered state—such as dreaming, meditation, or intoxication—to communicate distress to the consciousness, when protecting the consciousness no longer works. Different stories, in the form of either feelings or visions, are locked in different locations in the body. How they become encoded there seems to be a highly individual thing.

That's why everybody needs to tell his or her story, because these stories are locked up in the body, unbeknownst to us. I found that about 75% of the information my body gave me in the Guided Imagery and Music process I undertook when I was healing from cancer was new to me, despite five years of therapy and some experience with meditation, yoga, and qigong. There were particular stories of war and war wounds and seafaring existences (more than one). I interpret these as past lives, having run across similar stories both in myself and in patients; other people might interpret them in other ways. In these experiences I found some plausible explanations for some unexplained quirks of mine.

Replacing the default with consciousness

We are designed with default responses to illness or trauma, largely unconscious, which are sometimes appropriate to the situation and sometimes not. Such pain and stress responses are meant to be short-term only, and when they become chronic, a disease state can be created. A simple example of a default response is holding your breath when in pain. Theoretically, you hold your breath to keep from moving the injured part and hurting it again, but this is probably the wrong thing to do after the acute stage has passed. Pain results from ischemia (not enough blood getting to the part), so if you continue to hold your breath, you'll make the pain worse. You can override the default response here by taking a deep breath to oxygenate the place that hurts.

I teach a simple form of biofeedback, derived indirectly from the experiments of Elmer Green, as described by Norman Cousins in *Head First.* Dr. Green taught cancer patients to raise the skin temperature of their hand by concentrating on it. I had two questions: What practical use can be made of this phenomenon, and why on earth should anyone wait to be diagnosed with cancer before learning this most basic life skill? Since pain is caused by ischemia, sending blood to the place that hurts not only relieves pain, but often solves the problem. A dirty little secret here: You don't have to be a yogi to do this. My cat knew how. Some people can do it immediately, and some require more practice. Some are not aware that they are doing it, even when they are. I either touch the spot in question or have the patients do it. All the hand does is show them where to direct their attention. If they don't feel it, even that's okay; envisioning the hand in place can be enough. I usually tell them to hold for a count of twenty or until they feel a change. I taught this at a healing service once. "A miracle!" someone said. "That pain I had went away." It is a miracle—an everyday one, commonplace, reproducible.

When I was in chiropractic school, I was experimenting with this, which I refer to as "sending." "How do you know you're directing blood to the area?" a resident asked me. So the next time there was a blood drive, I tested it, while my blood was being drawn, by "sending" to the arm with the needle in it. The nurse commented that the bag was filling awfully fast and became concerned that I was bleeding too much when she took the needle out. "Silly me," I said to myself; "I forgot to shut it off." So I directed the circulation to the other arm in order to stop the bleeding. During a visit, I told this story to my sister and my niece. After I left, my niece had a nosebleed that she couldn't stop. My sister said to her, "Send to your feet." The nosebleed stopped.

Six

Simple, Profound Truths

I have found there to be basic principles that apply to the healing process.

- If there has been illness or trauma, there needs to be repose and comfort.
- If there has been tearing down, there needs to be building up.
- If there has been starvation, there needs to be food—food as nature created it, not as chemists synthesize it.
- If people have been silenced, they need to speak their truth.
- If they have experienced devastation, they need hope.
- If they have been rendered powerless, they need to reclaim control of their lives. If they are bewildered, they need to understand.

Doesn't that seem simple and self-evident? Apparently not—at least not in the way allopathic medicine handles cancer today.

Isn't it time to bring kindness back to medicine?

.

PART II

My Journey

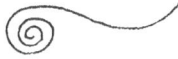

Seven

Don: "You'll be too late to help me"

February 1980-December 1987

This is an account of my discovery that I, even with my rudimentary training at the time, could take someone temporarily out of pain who was suffering from a serious, possibly terminal, condition. I think this is also when I unwittingly set the intention to find a way to help people with a diagnosis of cancer. The events in this piece took place long before the rest of my story.

My friend and I were talking about Local One. Stage Employees' Local #1, IATSE, is the stagehands' local in New York City, where I apprenticed and worked for twelve years before going to chiropractic college. In 1975 I took and passed the apprentice exam, the first year that the exam was open to women, becoming the first woman to hold a card in Local #1. I served my apprenticeship at CBS-TV in Special Effects and received my full membership card in January 1980.

I told my friend of the many colleagues and mentors I had who were about twenty years older than I, and how I am seeing now their importance in helping me along my path. The evening of that conversation I realized that Don died in December 1987, twenty years before. I felt him contacting me to remind me that he was also a part of this story.

Gentleman Don

My first job after getting my full union card was at Madison Square Garden, running a spotlight for the Ice Capades. I had almost no experience—let's modify that—none whatsoever. One thing about running an ice show is that everything moves extremely fast. The sixteen spotlights in the Garden are inside the ceiling above the ninth floor (the ice itself is on the fifth). As the skaters move up and down the ice, the size of the spot changes, and color changes are called while the lights and the skaters are moving. We would run this show without rehearsal.

Several of the spotlight operators were old-timers in the business (at least in comparison to me), who helped me figure out how to run the lamp. Don was one, and he and I became friends. We would figure out during the morning show where we were going for lunch, which became a ritual of ours.

Don's father was known as "Doc" Kurtis. This was not merely a nickname or a courtesy title; he had been a chiropractor and massage therapist since 1922. My first chiropractic table belonged to him, and I still have copies of his chiropractic and massage licenses. Chiropractors were not licensed in New York State until 1963, and Doc also worked as a stagehand. He invented the Kurtis wrench, a tool once used to tighten the yoke on a certain type of spotlight. So Don was brought up in the business. He had an engineering degree from Stevens Institute of Technology but the births of his children had necessitated his going back to being a stagehand. He was not really content with being one.

Don was ever the gentleman and enjoyed squiring the ladies around town, first me, and later, me and Gretchen. He liked classical music and jazz and introduced me to an early recording by Wynton Marsalis. We would stroll around in the vicinity of the Garden between shows; on other occasions we would go to the Tavern on the Green and sit outside munching on crudités. He always enjoyed showing me new and interesting places to eat. "It's easier to adopt you than to marry you," he said. I still remember his taking my hand as we crossed the street, just as my father used to.

Don and Zita got married in 1982 and bought a house in Chester, near the Goodspeed Opera House, where I went to visit. Not long after that, he was diagnosed with lung cancer, which could have been caused by asbestos in the ceiling at the Garden; there was also a possibility that it might have been related to outgassing from the lamps on the spotlights. Another of our co-workers developed a brain tumor a year or two later. Thus began years of lawyers and depositions. The wheels of the law ground extraordinarily slowly, and Don became unable to work, so the money ran down and they moved from one smaller house to another. A settlement was finally reached—after his death.

I had introduced him to the works of Lewis Thomas, *The Lives of a Cell* and *The Medusa and the Snail*, which were an important early influence on my thinking about things medical and biological. I admired Dr. Thomas as a scientist who could actually write, intelligently and wittily, who drew meaning from his experiences and observations that he was able to translate into everyday life. It was in his books where I first found out that our mitochondria, the tiny "power plants" inside every cell, do not have the same genetic material as we do, but instead are symbionts, which means they perform their energy-creating function for us, while we provide them with food, protection, and the ability to move around. I found this fascinating. Don found the books fascinating, as well, and took it a step further, entering into correspondence with Dr. Thomas.

If any creature offers you love

Before he got sick, there had been an undercurrent of anger and discontent in Don. After the diagnosis, this began to shift, which I understand better now. I still remember one conversation we had while walking along 57th Street. He said to me, "If any creature in the universe offers you love, accept it."

In 1984, I began to think about going to chiropractic school. He asked if I might consider medical school; I said I thought not. He thought that if I went to medical school I might be able to do something about cancer—"But you'll be too late to help me."

I still remember an idyllic visit with him and Zita, during which we swam in the Connecticut River, went sailing with his neighbor, and docked at the Gelston House next door to the Goodspeed Opera House for lunch. Zita had clams, to which I am allergic, and I had shrimp, to which she was allergic. Don had had lung surgery not long before and was in pain. I worked on him later that afternoon and was able to take him out of pain for two hours. I will never forget that.

Our last visit to Don and Zita was in the fall of 1987. I had no idea how sick he was by this time—"He didn't want to worry you girls," Zita said. We actually ended up going there for a foolish reason—I had bought a tire nearby on the way to Nova Scotia during the summer that turned out to be defective, so I was going to get a refund for it. Later I recognized this as the universe making sure that we would see Don again before he died.

Gretchen and I had a phone call from Zita in December of 1987, telling us that Don had collapsed while drinking a glass of chocolate milk and died on the way to the hospital. "We have to go there," Gretchen said. Zita, being from California, had no family in the area. We stayed a few days and helped out with the seemingly endless paperwork and arranging that someone's exit from the world entails. We also washed out the glass of chocolate milk that was still sitting on the counter.

In the fall of 1988, Karen S. and I were riding along the shore road near Hammonasset Beach, near Don's last house. He rode in the car with us in spirit for a bit, and left as we passed near the house. "My girls will take care of each other," he said. I told Zita about it later. We agreed that is exactly what we might have expected him to say.

Eight

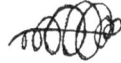

Jean: The Meanings of Pain

December 1996-October 1998

A psychic once told Jean that her life would change on December 13, 1996. That was the day she called me.

I had opened my chiropractic practice in April 1995, so I had been in practice for less than two years at the time I met Jean. Though of course I did not know it at the time, the intense, ten-year process of treating her would be crucial to my ability to heal myself. In working with Jean I would also experience, for the first time, cleaning up the damage done by the conventional medical profession, something I would have to do time and time again over the years.

Together, Jean and I learned many of the basic principles that now inform my healing work.

You'll see why as you learn her extraordinary story.

I had met Jean the previous August, when I was substituting for her regular chiropractor, something I did not deem a success and never attempted again. "Jean liked the way you worked on her neck," the receptionist told me.

In December, after having severe headaches that just seemed to get worse when she went to the chiropractor, she finally told him that she was going to try the low-force style of work that I did. "It's your only hope," he said. That day she had had to stop halfway on the ten-mile trip home because the headache was so bad.

Walked in, wheeled out

Jean came in to see me on December 14, and so our work began. On that first visit I focused mainly on the headache, which did abate to some extent. She gave me a history on this initial visit, of course, but it was to take quite a while for me to begin to understand the complexity and enormity of her condition. She had worked for many years at the Wassaic, New York Developmental Center as a developmental aide, caring for clients with mental retardation and other developmental disabilities. A few months before her most recent injury, in 1977, she had received her nursing degree and had been promoted.

There had been several injuries, which for Workers' Comp purposes boiled down to two. The last and most severe of these, the one that caused her disability, occurred in 1977, when she was attacked by a client who slammed her knees to the floor and her back and neck against a bed. (No, 1977 is not a typo.) When she first came to me, she walked on two crutches for short distances and used a wheelchair for long ones.

She had had nine surgeries on each knee, which culminated in bilateral patellectomies (removal of both kneecaps). Constant severe pain in the low back had been treated unsuccessfully by nerve blocks and an assortment of drugs until, in 1986, it was finally found that there was a bone chip floating around in her low back. This was surgically removed. "I walked into the hospital," she says, "and left in a wheelchair. In physical therapy they had me putting pegs in holes. It was ridiculous. I told them I wasn't a stroke patient and what I really needed to learn was how to transfer to and from the wheelchair, and if they weren't going to teach me that, I was going to check out of the hospital. That's what I did. I stopped at the *Poughkeepsie Journal* on the way home and worked my paper route."

A painful problem: Buprenex

Jean and her doctors had struggled for years to find the right pain medication. She had previously tried many different medications and then a morphine pump, until, one day, she drove back from her chiropractic appointment in an ice storm and couldn't remember the trip. This frightened her. Eventually, in 1992, her pain management specialist settled upon Buprenex (buprenorphine), an agonist/antagonist morphine derivative, which means that Buprenex would relieve pain without producing a high.

The effectiveness of this medication, like many others, depends on the mode of delivery. The most effective method of delivery is a central line into the heart, so that the medication goes directly into the bloodstream. After the medication is delivered, it is followed by heparin to prevent clotting, and then cleaning of the line with saline solution. When we began, Jean was in severe enough pain that she was considering having a central line put in again, but we decided to wait and see. She was giving herself four intramuscular shots a day, which does not provide the degree of relief given by delivery through a central line. As of that time, there was no oral form of Buprenex. Now there is one, called Subonex—but it has only been in existence since 2004. It is less effective than the injectable form.

"I was like a pin cushion," she says. "I had been scheduled for surgery to put in the central line in October, but then Father went into the hospital and I canceled the appointment. Father died at Thanksgiving." Prior to that, she had had a central line put in on three separate occasions, and on all three occasions had developed septicemia. The first time it went for a year before being diagnosed, because nothing showed up on the lab work. In the beginning I had no idea about all of this. It was a measure of her desperation that she would even consider a central line again.

Fifteen minutes is enough...?

Because someone once decided that the average chiropractor works for fifteen minutes, that is the limit to the compensation Workers' Comp pays chiropractors in New York State. Jean's previous chiropractor did what they paid him for, once to three times a week. I quickly determined that this wasn't going to do the job, and had her come in three times a week; we spent one-and-a-half to two hours each visit.

She was out of the wheelchair in six months.

I quickly found that Jean was intelligent, highly motivated, and read voraciously on many topics related to healing. In one of the early visits, she showed me a passage in a book about Tai Chi and asked if it might be helpful. I had taken a Tai Chi class in 1995 and thought it would be excellent. So I wrote out a set of exercises, adapting them for use in a seated position. I still give the same set to patients so I can tell them that the patient for whom I wrote them is now walking without crutches, although she could not stand unsupported when I first gave them to her.

"We're going to change our strategy," I said. "Up until now, you've been using the drugs to block pain, and it has been necessary, but now I want you to bring the pain to consciousness so you can work with it. If it is buried, it cannot be healed." We also talked about supplementation. Her other chiropractor had put her on calcium; I added magnesium. She told me the next time she came in that the magnesium had cleared her constipation problem. This makes sense. Calcium tonifies; magnesium relaxes. They work together. Recent research alleging that calcium is ineffective in treating osteoporosis is meaningless because magnesium was not included in the protocol. Milk of magnesia is a well-known laxative.

"I also have these blackouts sometimes," Jean said, and so I showed her the chapter in *Dr. Wright's Guide to Healing with Nutrition* relating to this type of problem, which listed a number of supplements she could try. She still uses several of these, but bromelain is her favorite and she swears by it. Bromelain is a digestive enzyme derived from pineapple. Taken with meals, it is a digestive aid; taken between meals, it is an antiinflammatory and helps with bruising. It is a favorite for dealing with sports injuries.

Jean's Catch-22

Jean was in a Catch-22 situation when we started. Because of the disc problems, it was imperative that she walk. Sitting was the worst thing she could possibly do, but her knees were so unstable that she couldn't walk. The removal of the patellas meant that there was nothing to prevent the knees being twisted and possibly reinjured. The knees would not even let me touch them. Instead, I worked with the energy field around them, which was interrupted at the knees.

So how could we get the knees working again? They hadn't worked as knees in quite a long time and had forgotten what they were supposed to do. I had been doing some experimenting with magnets and suggested Jean put them over where the kneecaps had been. She asked me why. I came up with some sort of rationale that sounded pretty good, but that wasn't the reason at all. I had been given an inner message to suggest the magnets, but didn't know Jean well enough yet to admit it.

In April 1997 I attended a seminar on the patella at NYU that only cost $50 because it was sponsored by a drug manufacturer. It was given by surgeons, and the vendors' display in the lobby had fascinating surgeons' tools, jigs, prosthetic knee parts, and so on. This brought home to me how much of surgery is carpentry, and also how difficult it could be to know exactly where one was while in the middle of an operation. I am profoundly grateful that I am not a surgeon. As it is, if I confuse my left with my right I only waste a little time.

On the way down to the city in the train, I sat with the reports of Jean's eighteen knee surgeries and read them. I was in tears when I finished.

Some prominent surgeons in the field were at the NYU seminar, and I took advantage of the opportunity to ask them if they had any suggestions on how to treat a patient with bilateral patellectomies.

"We don't do that any more," one said.

Would it be possible to put in a prosthesis for the patella?

No. There wasn't enough of the original structure left.

I spoke to the physical therapist who had done a presentation on rehabilitation and asked his advice.

"I've never seen a patient with bilateral patellectomies," he said.

I was on my own.

Jean walks without crutches

That April was remarkable for two other reasons—the addition of two major characters to my practice. Shirley started with me on a Saturday. I remember this so well because she was in trouble with low back pain after her first adjustment, and I had a couple of panic calls from her on the following day, Sunday. She couldn't get out of bed, so I made a house call. Jean was staying with her that day, and I watched as Jean walked down the hall carrying a chair, wearing braces on both legs, but using no crutches. I had never seen her walk without crutches before.

I successfully got Shirley ambulatory, and early the next week she came for a followup visit. While she was there, two children came by, saying they had to move and needed to find a home for their cat, and would I take him?

Mr. Moose, my previous cat, the last of my New York City cats, had just died in August, and since then I had been staying at Sharon's. I had no intention of getting another cat at this point.

The universe decided otherwise.

The cat wasn't a he. She was a she, but at least they were correct in that she had been fixed, so kittens were not an issue. She was a gorgeous longhair. They called her Willy; I changed that to Wilhelmina. After only one night of hiding under the furniture, she was jumping up on the table and adjusting patients as if she were born to it. She also enjoyed a secret life, attracting a multitude of admirers as she held court in the front window.

Jean progressed rapidly. We soon had her down to two shots a day. The wheelchair went into storage in June. On every visit, I ask the patient to fill in a pain drawing so that I can track progress. On an outline drawing of the body, he or she shades in the areas of pain and assigns a number from 0 to 10 to indicate the intensity of the pain. The character of her pain drawings had changed since the beginning, and they were now so accurate that I could have adjusted from them with no other information. This is highly unusual. Most people will simply put an x, a circle, or a single line on the spot that hurts and are not aware of other areas that may be involved. The reduction of pain medication, along with a lot of hard work, was allowing her much more body awareness than she had had before, and she was becoming mentally sharper. I was also noticing as we worked that I might feel an odd pain here or a buzz there on myself.

While working with other patients on other occasions, I had felt these sensations but ignored them. This began happening often enough with Jean, however, that I started asking her whether she was feeling the same sensations as I, and she would say, yes, her left foot felt as if it were in a bucket, or her right hand was numb, or yes, she had a pain in her lower right ribs. Although I pick up the sensation through my hands, I will feel the pain in the same part of my body as she is feeling it in hers, with the same quality. I assume that I do not feel the same intensity, so I usually have to ask if what I am doing is so painful that I need to stop.

We encounter Lyme disease

I had "read" other people in this manner before, but this is when I really learned to pay attention to what I was being told.

Then, one day in July, Jean got what turned out to be a tick bite and came down with a full-blown case of Lyme disease. I suspect that years of using pain medications may have impaired her immune function. The constant pain, which we had managed to reduce to a level of 6/10 on the pain scale, became a 10/10, much more relentless and unresponsive to anything I did. It took on a life of its own and felt alien, not like part of her at all. She was prescribed the usual course of doxycycline, but as soon as she went off it, the symptoms returned. She was put on another course and the same thing happened.

In September, Jean and I went together to the Green Nations Gathering, an herbal conference. Noteworthy at that conference were presentations by herbalist and biochemist Hart Brent on ehrlichiosis—a tick-borne disease that often appears as a co-infection with Lyme— and Dr. Rosita Arvigo, a naprapath, on Mayan Uterine Massage. Naprapathy is a system of manipulation bearing some similarity to chiropractic but gentler, originated by Dr. Oakley Smith. For many years, naprapaths were not licensed, and now naprapathy is taught only in the Chicago area. I did not attend Dr. Arvigo's intensive, but bought the tape.

Jean hardly slept at all during the weekend of the herbal conference. I found out that this is quite common with Lyme, though I was not so familiar with it then. Nevertheless, she navigated around the rather rough terrain with only one crutch.

Healing prayer: letting the mind catch up

At the same time, Teresa had started going to the healing service at the Oratory of the Little Way in Gaylordsville, Connecticut, upon the recommendation of her pastor. I wasn't particularly interested in healing prayer but figured I couldn't say it didn't work if I hadn't tried it. Teresa would describe to us the three or four prayer teams in the corners of the church after the main service—"There has to be someone behind to catch if they rest in the Spirit," she said. This response to healing prayer was also known as "carpet time."

Jean slept soundly the night after we returned home from the conference. Teresa told us later that she had stood in as a proxy for Jean at the healing service and asked that she be able to sleep. This got our attention, and all four of us decided to go with Teresa to the healing service the next Tuesday. The guest preacher that day, from the Order of St. Luke, was reading a scripture on the subject of "Why do you want to be healed?" This got my attention also, as apparently it was as much a question in Jesus' time as in mine. I had heard Scripture, but never listened to it as an adult and found it entirely different this time.

We went quite regularly to the healing service. I experienced carpet time myself more than once. Nigel Mumford, the leader of the Oratory at the time, used to describe it as "heavenly anesthetic." I found that I was aware of what was going on around me but could neither speak nor get up until whatever was happening was completed. On one occasion, I got up off the floor and realized that my winter depression had lifted.

Jean found that she needed to wear her braces whenever she went up for prayer, because she might twist one of her knees and not be able to get up off the floor again. Nigel expressed the hope that someday she would walk into the church without her crutches. It is important to mention the Oratory here because I think the healing prayer made it possible for us to go on to the next step in her healing.

We struggled with Jean's Lyme disease through the rest of the fall and into the winter, with relapses occurring each time she went off the doxycycline. Obviously that wasn't working. The pain was unrelenting and unaffected by anything that I did. We had been moving along very quickly before that, but now our progress ground to a halt.

Finally, around January or so, she was put on another antibiotic, Ceftin, one of the cephalosporins. It was really nasty and gave all of her food a bad taste. Toward the end of the course, the alien quality of the pain was persisting. I observed that either the antibiotic wasn't working or she was having a bad reaction to it, and in either case she needed to stop it then and there. This worked. The cephalosporins are related to penicillin, to which she was allergic. This either didn't occur to me at the time or I didn't know about the penicillin allergy yet.

She had suffered quite a setback with the Lyme. *But I know that the universe provided the Lyme at that point because her physical healing had been progressing much faster than her mind and emotions could handle it.*

Then, in March, we started to progress again. I was working on her low back and felt the tissues part and meet again. That was all. I didn't pick up any pain. It was the tactile equivalent of watching a movie.

I was experiencing a playback of the back surgery.

One night, while I was lying in bed, I got the message that I was to reconnect Jean's body with her consciousness. I was intimidated by that, and gave some sort of "Who, me?" response.

"If you don't, who will?" was the answer.

These visions and impressions increased in intensity and frequency, and I started writing them down in a notebook. I soon realized that I needed to catch them soon after they occurred or they would be gone forever. They were often as evanescent as dreams. Sometimes I would recall something during the act of writing that I had forgotten.

The body speaks in the language of pain

When we began, Jean's pain had been a meaningless cacophony, as perceived by her and as felt by me. As time went on, it sorted itself out into several patterns, which I came to recognize as I felt them. Each type of pain was clearly related to a given theme or incident. There was the "bearing the burden" pattern across the neck and shoulders; this related to caring for her mother who had been an invalid since Jean was nine years old. When I first worked with the cranials, I felt a deep blackness across the lambdoidal suture on the back of the head. This was associated with the time a client had grabbed her from behind by her hair and slammed her head on the floor. As we worked, the deep blackness lessened, but this has always been a trouble spot. Ever since that injury, she had not been able to tolerate loud noise or music and has preferred to sit with her back toward the wall so no one could come up behind her. There was also the "garbage can" pain pattern, a band around the head. We called it that because it seemed as if the top of her head were a lid that was being lifted to let the garbage out.

There were also mechanical problems that were easy to explain, such as the rib pains that resulted from years of twisting to give herself the Buprenex shots, or the shoulder and wrist problems from years of crutch and wheelchair use. We were always working with these.

I have found that it is imperative to separate pain into its component parts in order to cope with it. Regardless of its primary cause, there will be different components, such as toxicity, nutritional deficiency, low oxygen due to muscle spasm or poor biomechanics, and emotional factors. For example, once I treated a patient for toothache pain. She was pregnant at the time and couldn't take any drugs. There was severe muscle spasm in the jaw, and when I released it, the pain went away. Did I get rid of the cavity that was causing the problem? Quite clearly not. Was the pain gone after treatment? Yes. Would it recur? Probably. The pain was caused by the muscle spasm, which in turn was caused by the body's universal tightening reaction to something it didn't like—the cavity.

At times I would get a feeling or see an image, would tell Jean what I saw and she would tell me what it was about. "You're running," I said one time, and she said, yes, she was running away from a rattlesnake in the barn. "Your ears are burning," I said another time. "Someone said something to you," and she said that one of the farmhands had made an embarrassing remark when she was in her early teens, so she had thrown a cow pie at him—and he never did that again. "You're riding something," I said another time, as I felt surges of energy running up and down her spine. She said, yes, it was Spot the cow, when she was about five years old—"She was my only friend."

Easter Sunday brought another change. A close friend left her husband and moved in with Jean. The relationship had ended with an incident of sexual abuse that was the last straw—"But you wouldn't understand," the friend said to Jean.

"Oh, yes, I would!" Jean replied.

Two knees, two voices

Toward the summer we decided on a surgical consultation about the condition of Jean's knees. They were still very unstable, and the old braces weren't preventing their twisting. The surgeon recommended a trial of physical therapy on the knees. Ultrasound was tried but it caused too much pain even at the lowest setting, so it was discontinued after only two treatments. The surgeon said that the joints were in good condition, so a total knee replacement didn't make sense at this time.

The knees, which up until that time had not communicated much with me, had quite a bit to say about all this. The right knee, which we called Baby, "spoke" to me as if it were about three years old. Jean had been boarded out at this age to some not very nice people who fed her nothing but oatmeal. The left knee was either nine or eleven years old, a bit of a smart aleck. We called her Sissy. Both of them made it clear that nobody was going to be doing any surgery on them, and that they didn't trust anybody to work with them except me.

Jean reassured the knees that nobody was going to do any surgery on them, and they calmed down, and it was from this time on that they became quite vocal. Baby, in particular, could be quite articulate and sophisticated at times for a three-year-old. Sissy prided herself on her strength and her ability to do almost anything; she was the one who took care of things. They insisted that we promise to treat them once a week.

When we began, Jean said she was only able to drive to the doctor's and the grocery store. This was changing rapidly. At the end of June, she and Teresa drove to Vermont to Fishnet, a healing conference with which Nigel from the Oratory was associated. Four or five days of intensive healing prayer, along with our work, began to break down years' worth of defenses for both Jean and Teresa and brought them closer. Around this time I had been beginning to suspect that there was more complexity to Jean's pain than the injuries alone would explain, severe and traumatic as they were. Bits of her story were beginning to leak out, first to Teresa and then to me.

One day, Jean and I were working, and I picked up such a bad headache that I had to stop. "Will this help?" she asked, taking off the crystal she was wearing and hanging it on the doorknob. It was labradorite, which she had picked up that day at a craft fair. Before I met Jean, she had become interested in making jewelry. "I began by stringing beads to distract myself from the pain," she said. "Then people started asking me to make jewelry for them." This led her to an investigation of the healing powers of stones and crystals. I had no familiarity with this at that time.

Only when she took off the crystal did my headache go away, enabling me to work again. I think the crystal had amplified the energy in her nervous system to the point that I could not tolerate it.

Medication down, clarity up

With the decrease in medication and corresponding increase in mental clarity, Jean became an avid student of feng shui. My old office had a lot of shortcomings, from the feng shui point of view. We couldn't do much about the structure and the lack of light and air, but Jean hung a crystal in the bedroom doorway and mirrors in the hall. The placement of the bed right opposite the doorway was poor feng shui, because the energy came directly into the room toward the bed. There was no other choice for placement of the bed, the room being small, so the crystal would fix that problem. The mirrors were intended to make it possible to see who was coming down the long hallway when I was working in one of the patient rooms. She also told me not to put the desk with the computer facing away from the door, or, if this was absolutely necessary, to place a mirror so that I could see anyone coming up behind me.

The week we made these small changes, three new patients came into the practice, seemingly from nowhere.

I have come to understand more about feng shui since these early days. It is less about the crystals and mirrors and other trappings than about arranging space to maximize efficiency and comfort in using it. The goal is to eliminate the three extra times one walks around the table looking for the thing one put down, and if you multiply these incidents over the course of days, weeks, or months, it makes a huge difference in both frame of mind and energy level. There is a certain type of irritation I sometimes feel, which I now recognize as a need to put some portion of the house in order. Furthermore, I also see this as a problem during times when the practice has been busy, and then the number of patients suddenly drops. This indicates that the feng shui is out of order again and I am tripping over myself.

I had seen an influx of Workers' Comp patients in 1997 and 1998, necessitating more paperwork. Teresa became valuable doing insurance work in the office and took over where Sharon had left off in helping me deal with the insanity of Workers' Comp. Comp was very slow to pay; at one point they owed me $2400 for my work with Jean in the middle of the winter, and consequently I could barely scrape together the money to pay the oil bill. Teresa was good at the type of dogged persistence required to deal with insurance companies—"I just keep hitting redial," she said.

Also during this period, Jean and Teresa were helping Sharon out at Calsi's General Store. Jean was the queen of the co-op orders and used this to full advantage to explore a multitude of herbs and supplements and introduce us to them. Before she came to me, years of pain and being housebound had turned her into a recluse. At Calsi's, she learned once again how to interact with people, develop friendships, and become an important resource for the customers there. Teresa, naturally gregarious, also thrived while working at Calsi's.

Jean, Teresa, Shirley and I often met for supper at the Round Tuit. They were a tremendous support as the practice got busier and I needed more help just to keep going. They would pick up toilet paper at the dollar store, straighten up the kitchen, and generally help out wherever it was needed. They usually knew what had to be done, and did it before I thought to ask. Jean, an expert bargain shopper, found me my fax machine and passed on her computers to me each time she upgraded. They had all joined the Ladies' Auxiliary of the Wassaic Fire Department and were excited about getting their uniforms for the upcoming parade season. I went to the parades to watch them march, or drive, in the case of Jean and Teresa.

We had become The Crew.

"Because of you, I cannot hide"

As spring went into summer, my work with Jean became ever more intense, as her body had more messages for me. We could never stay on the T7 vertebra long enough to make a difference. She told me that she had had a hysterectomy some years back; one ovary had been removed due to an extremely painful ovarian cyst. "I told the doctor he was going to have to remove the other one, too," she said, "and he said no. But a couple of weeks later he had to. I was full of endometriosis; they had to scrape off my intestines. I think that might have happened as a result of the first surgery." I thought she might have some feeling of regret about this, but she said she was glad to be rid of it. It was a while before it came out, but I was beginning to suspect a history of sexual abuse in Jean's past.

And so there was, much more intense and long-standing than I ever suspected. Bits of it began to leak out in her conversations with Teresa, who then would sometimes leak them to me, so I would have some indication of what we were in for. Frequent trips to the Oratory and healing conferences kept the flow going, so that Jean could process the things her body was telling her. "I vowed that no one would ever know about the sexual abuse," she said. In the early days, she wore her hat down low over her eyes so that it was difficult to see her face. This was beginning to change. "Because of you, I couldn't hide any more," she said.

Things occurring in Jean's present would bring up a body memory. For example, she once had a dental infection. As I was standing behind her, working on her cranials and neck, her body was reminded of one of the three incidents of septicemia. I kept receiving playbacks of this for two solid weeks and urged her to get the dental work done. Finally I felt the tug as the catheter was pulled out from her heart. It knocked me off my feet.

The practice was getting busier. Up until sometime late in 1998, I had been teaching the Tai Chi set to all the patients, which had the benefit of making sure that I did it consistently and kept a modicum of sanity in my life and in the practice. Sanity, however, was beginning to erode. There were many nights when I sat at the Round Tuit with the Crew, a stack of seven patient files in front of me, and even after eating supper I could barely marshal the brains to fill them out. "Who were all these people, anyway?" I would ask, and I was only half joking. Usually a muffin at the end of supper was necessary to bring my blood sugar up to the point where I could write the files. The number of Comp patients had increased, so I was working harder, yet making less money, and from time to time I was having to prod the carriers to pay my bills, which sometimes worked and sometimes didn't.

Sometime subsequently, I don't remember when (maybe in 2001), Jean accidentally received a bill from the drug company for $3,000 for one month's worth of Buprenex. She called the company to ask about it, and they said they had negotiated this rate with her insurance carrier in September 1996. Since that time, we had reduced the use of Buprenex by 50%, but the drug company was still charging the same price, so she asked about it. "Sometimes we win, sometimes we lose," the drug company representative said.

I was seeing her three times a week, at $27.11 per visit (this rate went into effect in September 1997 and has not changed since!). This comes to $81.33 per week, a maximum of $406.65 in a five-week month for chiropractic care, without which she would not be walking today. Yet I have had to have periodic wrangles with the carrier to get them to approve this, while they would pay $3000/month for Buprenex without a murmur. As of this writing, in 2008, the carrier will pay for four treatments a month, totaling $108.44.

Nine

Doc: The Student Is Ready, the Teacher Appears

November 1998-May 2001

Doc was present in spirit during the gong meditation in yoga class last week. He knows that I am writing a book and says he wants me to tell his story. It is a long and tumultuous story, and I was only in on the last chapter. I had not felt his presence so strongly since he appeared in a dream to say goodbye, three weeks after his passing. I should not be surprised; we had agreed to contact each other after he passed. He is as good as his word.

Herbert Spencer Feldman, DC, ND was referred to me by a former patient of both of ours. Doc told me he had not been adjusted in four years, which was nearly unthinkable for someone who had been born into, lived, and breathed chiropractic. His father was a chiropractor and they had worked together for many years.

"Your liver is vibing red" were the first words Doc spoke to me. I had been eating too much beef and potatoes, and had recently decided to go off them after experiencing digestive trouble, which I had never had before. Doc said he had been able to see auras since he was thirteen years old, and could also see organs. My liver was indeed vibing red. He was right.

It was certainly not the last time he would be right.

How would I describe Doc at that first meeting? "Unprepossessing" would be as good a word as any. He was slight in build, no taller than I, with white hair and a receding hairline, and was missing most of his teeth. I had heard rumors about him since I first moved into town. Some warned me against being seen with him. Yet people who had been his patients told me he had saved them. At least one person told me that the only reason he was able to walk was because of Doc.

I decided to try to ignore the rumors and negativity, in order to see for myself, which was one of the best decisions I ever made. And what if I hadn't? The cancer might have taken an entirely different, more virulent course without Doc's medical intuition and guidance. I might (who knows?) have given in to pressure and had a hysterectomy. And this book would not exist.

Doc vs. the medical establishment

Doc's life had been full of harshness and injustices. He had practiced with his father and had not married until his fifties. His wife had been a patient and they married not long after his father's death. She had spent her early childhood in London during the Blitz and was manic-depressive. "She needed me as much as I needed her," Doc said. For the first five years he was able to control her illness without lithium.

As time went on, her condition worsened and he could no longer control it. He was under a lot of pressure to treat her according to the state of the art at the time, which consisted of institutionalizing her and giving her Thorazine, which ran contrary to everything he believed. This drug is infamous for its most visible effect, the "Thorazine shuffle." It also makes coherent thought and speech impossible, which makes the patient docile. As was mentioned in the previous chapter, communication between the body and the consciousness is necessary for healing either physical or psychic trauma. Everyone needs to tell his or her story. Doc knew that as long as his wife remained in a Thorazine-induced stupor, it would be impossible for her to get well.

She died after hitting her head in a freak accident. What may never have been mentioned in the courtroom during Doc's trial was that she had had twelve electroshock treatments before Doc had ever met her. He did not know that at the time they married, but found it out later. Doc and I talked about this, and it seemed logical to both of us that her head and brain might have been made more susceptible to injury as a result. I surmise that, if someone without a history of shock treatments had experienced a similar injury, she might simply have walked away, rubbing the bump on her head.

Doc could be brusque, which was not helpful when it came to communicating. When he was working and information came through, it came tumbling out in a flood that he could not control or modulate to suit the sensibilities of his audience, and he offended people at times. Had circumstances been different, we could have worked well together, since I could understand what he was saying and interpret it for others.

A doctor without a license

Adjusting Doc on that first day was somewhat like adjusting a brick wall. He said he had recently been released from prison, where he had been for two or three years, and now was out on parole. He had not been put in jail for murder, as several people in town had told me. I find it probable that the criminal negligence charge stemmed from his reluctance to institutionalize his wife. He told me that the charges had had nothing to do with his practice of almost fifty years. Nevertheless, the State Education Department had revoked his license. Later on, we investigated the possibility of applying for reinstatement. This would have involved a payment to the State Education Department of seven hundred fifty dollars and submitting ten affidavits as character references, three of which would have to be signed by other chiropractors. It seemed to me that this was a humiliating process.

"Your body is not your own," he said about prison, where he had no control over his diet; neither did he have any control over the type of treatment he received. During his incarceration he had developed prostate trouble, which they had treated with medication (Proscar) to which he was allergic. He described walking in chains, itching all over, while having to take this medication.

Those who do not normally take drugs will often be much more sensitive to them than other people, and doctors may tend to overdose such people. "The only kind of cranberry juice I could get in prison was loaded with sugar," he told me. Cranberry juice used for urinary tract problems should be unsweetened, as sugar will aggravate the problem. Sugar will also feed cancer. Left to his own devices, Doc might never have taken a drug at all, but instead might have focused on improving his nutrition.

He had no access to the herbs, supplements, and chiropractic care he would normally have used, so he was in poor condition when he came home. The prostate trouble had turned out to be cancer, which he said ran in his family.

He also had a heart condition, a result of the rheumatic fever he had had when he was ten years old. This had become exacerbated while he was in prison.

To make matters worse for Doc, construction on his house had been begun but not completed while he was away, so the home he returned to was a shambles. Court expenses had eaten up almost all of his savings. Medicare would not kick in for six months to a year after his release, so he had to pay all of his medical expenses out of pocket. He made some attempts at finding work, but was always turned down because of the felony conviction. The need to urinate every forty-five minutes limited the type of work he could look for. I remember buying him a tank of cooking gas one month.

Doc said that, though he had been able to see auras and organs with about 80% accuracy before going to prison, his accuracy was currently reduced to 50%. So far as I was concerned, he was seeing accurately, sick as he was, even before the first time I adjusted him.

"The friend who referred you to me said you were a *mensch,*" Doc told me. He also said that my hands reminded him of his father's—a very high compliment, and I took it as such. After I adjusted him he would check his vision on the patterns of the ceiling tiles and let me know when it had cleared. I always adjusted him before he adjusted me, to insure that he'd have the energy to work on me. His hands were strong but not rough, and he showed me a number of techniques that I still use to great effect, and some others for which my hands simply aren't strong enough.

The first two or three times we met, I tried adjusting him before supper, but I found that I was exhausted and almost feverish
as a result. So we established the ritual of meeting for supper on
Tuesdays and Fridays, and would work after that. Doc was a
great talker, so I had to learn to fill out my patient files while
talking about something entirely different during supper.

Radiation: Is this "healing?"

I had only been seeing him for a week or two when the radiation
treatments began; he was scheduled for a series of thirty-six.
Kathleen or another friend would drive him over to New Milford,
about forty minutes away, five times a week. My witnessing the
results left me with the unfavorable opinion of radiation I have
today, for the following reasons:

1. The radiation didn't halt the progress of the cancer, and
   may have sped it up.
2. It caused redness and irritation—that is, burns—on his
   face and on his legs. The skin remained hypersensitive
   for a long time.
3. It sapped his energy.
4. I suspect it may have also caused burns to his intestine
   and bladder, adding diarrhea to the painful urination he
   already had.
5. It may have caused the metastasis that ultimately killed
   him. Radiation can cause alterations in genetic material,
   possibly creating the very problem it is supposed to
   solve. The stated goal of radiation is to create free radicals, which is the very outcome one is trying to avoid in
   any other circumstance.

Was radiation really necessary or useful? It was not palliative. It did not halt the progress of the cancer. It did not improve Doc's quality of life. It created other problems. Therefore, so far as I am concerned, the answer is a resounding No.

"I'll know things are bad when I can't drive around on the lawnmower any more," Doc used to say.

His vitality went down. Riding the lawnmower got more tiring. Skin on his legs and face was reddened and painful. Then the diarrhea began, a side effect of radiation. He was already having to stop whatever he was doing to urinate every forty-five minutes before the diarrhea began, as well. Was the radiation improving Doc's quality of life? Definitely not, though it produced the desired effect of keeping his PSA down. (PSA, or prostate-specific antigen, is a blood marker used to monitor prostate cancer. It becomes elevated if the prostate capsule is broken, for example, by a tumor.)

Even before Doc began the series of radiation treatments, I was concerned about dehydration and was trying to get him to drink more. He wouldn't, however, because he said it made him urinate more, and urination was painful. This was another one of those Catch-22 situations, like the one with Jean's knees and back. Looking back on it, and applying my subsequent experience, I think it's possible that one factor contributing to the urinary frequency was inadequate hydration, as I think the kidneys were struggling to do their job of eliminating toxins without adequate water to work with. I've noticed myself that, if I am not well hydrated, urination may be frequent but scanty. Doc liked drinking coffee, which also may well have contributed to the bladder irritation and the poor hydration. The coffee probably did give him some energy and some comfort.

I suspect that one of the factors in the development of cancers may be chronic dehydration, since lymphatic flow is suboptimal in this case and flow of nutrients into—and waste products out of— the cells is not efficient. This is also a likely factor in the development of arthritis and other degenerative diseases. As people grow older, the sensation of thirst seems to become less and less reliable as an indicator of the need for water. Once thirst occurs, dehydration is already established.

High price of a low PSA

Radiation was the first of a series of generally painful and useless medical interventions Doc underwent. He was once put on an antibiotic that made him stiff all over. (One of the side effects of this medication, according to the *Physicians' Desk Reference*, is rupture of tendons. I recently heard about a former patient who suffered a rupture of the Achilles tendon after long-term use of this drug and will need to be in a brace until it heals.) As a chiropractor, I can tell you that the kind of stiffness caused by a drug is quite different from stiffness due to natural causes—there is an inexorable, unyielding quality about it, and it takes a titanic effort for the practitioner to communicate with the body through it—it is almost impossible. This experience with Doc is what taught me that I cannot fight a drug when working on a patient.

Radiation had made Doc's dehydration worse. Also, it did not prevent—and indeed its burning and scarring could have contributed to—obstruction of the urinary tract by the prostate tumor, so for a while he had to have a catheter.

This was painful and nasty and not a long-term solution. So the urologist suggested, and ultimately performed, a transurethral resection of the prostate, or TURP. This procedure consists of threading a tool with a small loop of wire at the end up through the penis into the urethra and heating the wire to burn out the obstruction, while the patient is under anesthesia. The obstruction was therefore replaced with incontinence, which plagued Doc for the rest of his life. Urination remained painful. Of course it would.

But the PSA remained low!

The combination of diarrhea and incontinence would have made housekeeping difficult enough for a healthy person, and by this time Doc was definitely not healthy. He needed home care. Again, I was too pressured with other problems to begin to address this one, and I had not yet acquired the experience I was later to have in coping with my mother.

What would have helped Doc? The Gerson Therapy, almost certainly. Doc introduced me to the Gerson therapy, which was originated by Max Gerson, MD, and has been around since the 1930s. Gerson determined that all cancers arose from problems with the liver and the digestion, and therefore his therapy is systemic in nature rather than local. His approach involves addressing the metabolism of the entire organism, rather than removing or irradiating an "offending" part. The extensive use of fresh fruits and vegetables provides a great deal of potassium and works to right the sodium-potassium balance that Gerson believed was faulty in all cancers. The use of salt is outlawed.

Maintaining this therapy would have been a full-time job, and it would be impossible for Doc to do it on his own.

Better without an MD?

The Edgar Cayce material had another helpful solution to offer: the castor oil pack, a mainstay of the Cayce protocols. If, as Gerson maintained, cancer begins in the liver and the digestion, we could have begun with the packs. Thinking about it subsequently, I was puzzled as to why Doc himself did not suggest this, either for himslf or for Kathleen, as he had worked with the Cayce material for so many years. A possible answer would emerge later.

Essiac, an herbal formula introduced by Rene Caisse, RN, was derived from an original formula used by the Ojibway tribe. It contains sheep sorrel, burdock root, slippery elm bark, and turkey rhubarb root. These herbs are digestive aids and/or immune system builders. Doc had a book on Essiac, which I found after he died. Earl Mindell, in *Earl Mindell's Herb Bible*, states that "The typical tribal medicine man was as well-equipped as any modern pharmacy to treat a wide range of medical needs, ranging from the common cold to birth control." And why would this not be so? Human beings evolved along with plants and were designed to eat, interact with, use, and be healed by them. Many plants contain compounds analogous to human and animal hormones that are of no particular benefit to the plant. One day Doc brought me some sheep sorrel from his yard. "It's full of Vitamin C," he said. This common weed, the primary anticancer ingredient in Essiac, is on the list of "Banned Invasive" plants in Connecticut.

So Doc knew, or had known about, the tools we could have used to cope with the cancer. However, I did not realize how much of his powers he had lost by this time. I was not yet experienced enough to trust my own. He was doing coffee enemas and Glyco-Thymoline enemas before he got too sick, so he was working on the detoxification part. But his nutrition was so poor that he had nothing to rebuild with.

I also suspect he would have been better off if he had never seen a medical doctor.

Now, as I acquire the experience I didn't have then, I come to understand Doc's anger and frustration more and more. I hope I can put my own similar feelings to good use for the benefit of all sentient beings, instead of turning inward and becoming self-destructive, as Doc did. I cannot afford to harbor righteous anger and powerlessness without a constructive outlet. The combination is deadly.

Doc "sees" my patients through me

In spite of it all, Doc stuck religiously to our schedule, and I was gratified to see his mind becoming sharper again after we had been working for a while. One evening, we were sitting in Four Brothers restaurant, finishing supper. I was working on the file of one of the female patients I had seen that day.

"She has a thyroid problem," Doc said to me across the table, though this patient had come to me because of a car accident. "I can see the calcification of the thyroid on the X-ray." The X-ray was across the street in my office at that time.

We went back to the office, put the patient's lateral cervical X-ray on the viewbox, and there, indeed, was the calcification of the thyroid. Doc explained that he saw these conditions through me, whether or not I consciously saw the same thing.

On another occasion, Doc said, "He has a neck problem." The patient in question had come to me with a knee injury, and nothing about his neck had turned up in the history I took. It turned out that the patient had had a C3/C4 fusion, which I didn't know at the time Doc saw it.

Doc had graduated from Palmer School of Chiropractic in Davenport, Iowa in 1950, entering a very different chiropractic world than the one I came into. Licensure did not occur in New

York State until 1963. "You could get arrested for taking a patient's blood pressure—that was considered 'diagnosis,'" Doc said. "You could get in trouble for telling a patient to take a bath." He had long held a resentment against the state licensing board for their treatment of blind chiropractors, of whom his father was one. "One reason I talk a lot," Doc said, "is because I had to be my father's eyes and describe to him what I saw. After forty years of being a chiropractor, they made my father take an exam. He was terrified."

Doc had a degree in naturopathy as well as chiropractic, and was interested in just about everything. Shortly before his father died, Doc had begun writing a book called *Health Without Medicine,* which was never finished, due to his father's death. I was unable to find the manuscript when I was going through his house after he died, so it is lost forever. I do know that whatever it contained was about thirty-five years ahead of its time.

What has happened to chiropractic?

Doc was a great proponent of many natural therapies, particularly hydrotherapy, the medicinal use of water in the treatment of some diseases. Many of his favorite therapies barely appear in the curriculum of chiropractic schools any more. "What are they teaching you?" he would sometimes ask with more than a hint of exasperation, and now, several years later, I am beginning to ask the same question myself. We get far more didactic information in chiropractic school now than he would have received in 1950—science is very different now—but we were taught almost nothing in the way of simple, practical, common-sense remedies. As an example, we were shown the anatomy involved with a hiatal hernia, but not how to diagnose or treat one. This I learned from Doc.

Between the two of us, did I get the better education? I'm not at all sure I did. It should be said right off that, unlike the medical profession, chiropractic is legally defined, at least in part, by those who do not understand it and in some cases are openly hostile, which is a huge problem right from the beginning. Since licensure, the chiropractic profession has tried to get on the insurance and third-party-payer bandwagon, and to a large extent has managed to do so, although we are still seriously underpaid by insurance companies, compared to MDs. This has had the unwanted effect of creating a "Bed of Procrustes" on which the profession is supposed to fit, in order to get insurance payments and not to intrude on the turf of the allopaths. In Greek mythology, the giant Procrustes made all travelers lie down on his bed. If they were too tall, he trimmed down their legs to fit; if they were too short, he stretched them until they were the right height.

In the early days, chiropractors had two decided advantages over MDs: They spent time with their patients, enough to get to know them and their problems, and they touched and healed them—with their hands! What a concept! With the increased prevalence of insurance and the "production" mentality, "practice management" strategists, and governmental insistence on ever more complicated documentation, many doctors are decreasing the time actually spent with patients. Insurance is so structured that it is easier to be paid for procedures than for time, and it is often stingy with payment, so the best way to make good money is by increasing volume. Adjusting up to a hundred patients a day is hard work, so some are getting on the gadget bandwagon, using "adjusting instruments," electric stim, ultrasound, and spinal decompression tables. These all have their usefulness, but cannot replace human touch. So the low-tech, high-touch niche that chiropractors used to occupy in the health-care marketplace is now being taken over by acupuncturists and massage therapists.

Giving up our power

The medical profession has also made a concerted effort over the years to restrict chiropractic and the other nonallopathic professions, even in cases where nonallopathic treatment is a more direct and better solution to the presenting problem than an antibiotic or a pain pill. As a consequence, some chiropractors have accepted the more limited "musculoskeletal practitioner" paradigm, in a (probably) vain attempt to gain respect and acceptance from the medical and insurance establishments. By doing this, I feel we have given up a great deal of our power as doctors in order to achieve second-class status as mechanics. This outlook ignores the original premise of chiropractic, that spinal dysfunction leads to nerve impingements, and that consequent nerve compression or irritation can cause overfunctioning or underfunctioning of related organs.

Unfortunately, research, which might otherwise be used to help "prove" the effectiveness of chiropractic, tends to be paid for by those with the deepest pockets, most often pharmaceutical companies, so the "results" will be slanted to make drugs look effective and natural remedies less so. The double-blind, randomized controlled trial, considered by many to be the " gold standard" of research, is totally impractical for testing any type of physical medicine modality. Even if this were not so, there are other elements to chiropractic besides the adjustment, such as nutritional and exercise counseling, and the effectiveness of the personality of the practitioner. This last element is almost impossible to quantify.

Government-funded studies tend to be focused on topics such as "the effectiveness of chiropractic in treating low-back pain." This, to my mind, is reinventing the wheel. How much more sense it would make to study the chiropractic treatment of pneumonia, otitis media (middle ear infection), irritable bowel syndrome, asthma, hiatal hernia, migraine, or premenstrual syndrome, all of which conditions have been known to respond well to chiropractic in clinical practice. Doc told me about relieving a patient's urinary tract obstruction on one occasion with adjustment and prostatic massage.

As it stands now, we, as chiropractors, have abandoned some of our trust in our own diagnostic and technical skills, and some of our trust in a Higher Intelligence at work within us, preferring instead to bow down before the tin gods, Research and Science. We, as people, have abandoned some of our trust in our own instincts, experience, and common sense, relying instead on the opinions of "experts." Sometimes, in giving too much importance to the "facts" they impose on us, we grow blind to the truth. I think it is too bad.

So back to my liver...

Doc had said my liver was vibing red. I had gained forty-five pounds since starting the practice in 1995, only three-and-a-half years earlier, the result of changes in diet and activity level and gradual hormonal shifts that had taken me by surprise. Doc put me on digestive enzymes and lots of B complex. I no longer got indigestion from spaghetti suppers—but I decided that I shouldn't eat spaghetti any more, either. I was approaching my fiftieth birthday. Menstrual periods were sparse and irregular, which so far as I knew up to that point was OK, though I thought maybe they'd slowed down sooner and more abruptly than they should have. I was feeling that it was time to incorporate more nutrition into the practice—"You're feeling your oats as a practitioner," Doc said.

I was treating up to twenty-three patients a week before Doc and I worked on my liver, spending an hour on average, and sometimes more, with each patient. That was all I could do without getting sick at that time. By the time Doc died, I could handle twenty-nine.

Should I have been seeing twenty-nine patients? *Definitely not.* I should have been using more of that energy for myself. I still have trouble with that idea.

Gerson had said that cancer begins with the liver and the digestion. With Doc, I began working on detoxifying the liver and improving digestion four years before the cancer was diagnosed, so while we did not manage to prevent it entirely, we lessened its impact to the point that I never got seriously ill from this supposedly "fatal" disease.

Also during this period, I was starting to see changes in my mother's functioning. She was coming to see me every week for lunch and for treatment. In the earlier days she brought lunch and arrived, if not on time, at least no more than a half-hour late. Later she'd come without lunch and might arrive three-quarters of an hour late. I would suggest supplements, but was not at all sure she was taking them. And she started engaging in a series of fender-benders, some of which I only found out about later.

The cost of "battling the system"

So, on the day my mother usually visited (Wednesday, so she could take her art class) I was scrambling to make lunch for her and myself, get her fed and get her treated before the next patient arrived. It didn't always work. As she became less functional, and as the practice accelerated, this became more difficult. Between 1997 and 1999 I acquired several Workers' Comp patients. I didn't realize at first that I was working a lot more, making a lot less money, and struggling harder to get paid.

Also during this period, I had a patient on Comp (another former patient of Doc's) who was on too many pain medications; furthermore, I was having trouble getting paid on this case, which was one of the most difficult I ever had. This situation kept getting worse, so in addition to everything else, I was often up until 3 a.m., writing letters to judges and lawyers to address current issues in the latest of an unending series of hearings, none of which ever seemed to resolve anything. So I was fighting both drugs (see comments above) and the Workers' Comp system to try to get this patient well. A decision was finally made in November 2000. We "won" the case. All this meant was that the carrier had to pay for two treatments a month, though the patient needed two a week. The carrier didn't feel inclined to pay the difference, so I was still stuck for unpaid bills.

Meanwhile, the roof in the office leaked in at least two places. A number of attempts to fix it were unsuccessful, and the mold in the place was getting worse. There had always been problems with getting enough light and air, and the building was uninsulated, so I had to figure out the precisely right temperature that would make the patient rooms comfortable but not too hot, while it was freezing everywhere else. The kitchen and the shower were in a large open room in the back, and the hot water tank held only ten gallons, so I learned to shower very quickly.

Doc was concerned about the effects of these conditions on my health, and so was I, but apparently not enough. By late 1998 I knew I had to move, without a clue about how this was supposed to happen.

The universe steps in

Once more the universe stepped in.

I received a piece in the mail from the Ken Roberts Company about a course in commodities trading that would cost $195. I kept reading the material over and over and could find nothing wrong with it. So, as a present to myself for my fiftieth birthday, I sent away for it. I studied it carefully for five months before making any investments. Early in 1999, at the Oratory's healing service, the guest preacher had words of knowledge for everyone who was there. He said to me, "Your financial prayers are being answered." I made some mistakes, and then in June paid $200 for two 310 gold call options.

Upon Sharon's suggestion, I began looking at houses for sale in town. Nothing available seemed quite right—too small, laid out wrong, or something. I had my first look at my current house on a 100-degree day in the summertime. It was exactly what I wanted, and I saw no way I could do it. My mother had offered me money for a down payment and then asked for it back so that she could buy a new car.

In October I cashed out the two gold options for $5600.

This paid off my last student loan. We celebrated with a student-loan burning bonfire at Sharon's house.

I looked at a number of "For Sale" signs on houses, as I walked past them in my turns around the block over that winter. Jean gave me the Carleton Sheets real estate course to look over, which was a tremendous help. It emphasized the importance of buying a property with an income, ideally enough income to support itself. Then Barbara said she'd be willing to rent space for her therapy practice in the house. There was a cottage in the back with a tenant already installed. In the spring, the house was still on the market; the tenant had not been able to make a bid that the owners would accept. I made an offer. They accepted.

All this time, when there were a number of stressful situations going on simultaneously, it was very satisfying and helpful to get together with Doc and be able to rant and rave about whatever was happening at the moment, especially as he understood the practice-related issues as no one else did. He was a tremendous support and was eager to pass on his fifty years' worth of knowledge as a master diagnostician and therapist.

I would be content to be one-quarter as good.

One day I was having some problem with my hand. Doc looked at it and worked on it. "Stabilize it with the other hand when you adjust it," he said.

"I can't. It's my hand."

"Oh. I forgot." We laughed with delight at the sheer silliness of it.

Doc helps me handle stress

On another occasion I was having trouble sleeping. I asked Doc about it. "I see you sleeping on your left side," he said. "Don't. Sleeping on your left side puts pressure on the heart." My quality of sleep improved when I took this suggestion. I became aware that I had a tendency to sleep on my left side when under stress.

Doc was a master at reading an X-ray, having served during World War II as an X-ray tech, studying tuberculosis. So he would look at films with me and point out findings such as the calcified thyroid mentioned above.

Ironically, and unfortunately, I did not yet have the experience to do the quality of healing work for Doc that I subsequently did for myself. But it was by working with and on Doc that I began to acquire both knowledge and confidence I would find so necessary later. "You're the doctor," he would say when I deferred to him on some question or other. I gradually learned somethng of his ability to see the whole person as well as the sum of the parts and to be aware not only of the organ in question but how it is influencing those around it. An example of this is a hiatal hernia putting pressure on the heart from below and thereby causing "heart" symptoms. More recently, I had a patient with a blood pressure of 200/100. There was a feeling of extreme fullness above the diaphragm—and below, extreme emptiness. What was the problem? In my opinion, though he was on a number of antihypertensive medications, the problem wasn't the heart at all. The muscle spasm in the diaphragm was so severe that it was pinching the abdominal aorta. I suspect that the blood pressure below that point was very low. I would not have known to look at the situation this way without Doc.

He asked one question and made one life-changing suggestion.

Enter Gerson and Cayce

The question: "Are you familiar with Gerson?" I was not. The Gerson Therapy, as I mentioned earlier, is a dietary therapy originated and developed by Max Gerson, MD, originally used in the treatment of tuberculosis and migraine, but later, and more famously, in the treatment of cancers. This therapy has been particularly successful in dealing with advanced, metastasized cancers that have not responded well to allopathic medicine. Mainstays of the Gerson Therapy are vegetable and liver juices given thirteen times a day, coffee enemas given five times a day, a vegetarian diet with a great deal of potassium, avoidance of sodium, castor oil taken orally, and speeding up the thyroid to aid in detoxification. Doc used to say that if he could have done Gerson, it would have saved his life. I think this is true. I found a copy of Gerson's book in a bookstore in Chicago in 1999 and began reading it.

The suggestion he made was, "I think you ought to take another look at the Edgar Cayce material." Edgar Cayce was the first and best-documented medical intuitive. He gave readings while in a trance state, describing detailed therapies, of which he had no knowledge while awake. The readings covered issues of body, mind, and spirit and described past lives of the patient and their influence on the current condition. My astrologer aunt had introduced me to Cayce in 1969. At that time I was mostly interested in the reincarnation stories, since I didn't have any health problems yet and didn't relate to that aspect of Cayce's readings. Around the time Doc made this suggestion, a patient had lent me her copy of Dr. Harold Reilly's *The Edgar Cayce Handbook of Healing through Drugless Therapy*. Another patient said he was familiar with Cayce, and we talked about it. I wondered if it was possible that everybody around me was familiar with the readings and I was the only one who wasn't.

Doc had made extensive use of the Cayce material in his practice. His friend, Dr. Aaron Steinberg, a fellow chiropractor in New York, had made use of chiropractic, Cayce modalities and other interventions to treat cancer successfully. "Diet was the most important," a former patient of his recounts. "There was nothing extreme in his recommendations. He suggested eliminating red meat, eating fish and chicken for protein, and eating a lot of raw fruit and vegetables. He used colonics, clay packs over the tumor, and Laetrile." [At one time, colonics were a part of the curriculum at National College of Chiropractic, but this has not been the case for more than twenty years.] "The clay was a special kind he got from Canada," she continued. "Before I met Aaron, he had gone to Japan to study acupuncture, and he used that as well. He put something over the breast that was the shape of an implant, and I think it vibrated. At first I saw him every day, then three times a week, then twice a week. The tumor was gone in seven months."

"Aaron took terrific chances with his license," Doc told me.

OK, Doc's suggestion about Cayce was the third such mention. This was a clear signal from the universe.

Our dinners twice a week at Four Brothers gave us ample opportunity to talk. Doc had a love for and interest in theology, and had studied Kabbalah. "The letter Aleph, as in *Adam,* stands for 'that which God gave you,'" he said. "Beth means 'house of .' Shin means 'the whole thing.'" And "Yeshua was a Jewish boy. He wasn't interested in starting a new religion; he was interested in reform." Our conversations led to my subsequent interest in and curiosity about gnosticism.

A woman at peace

Sometimes Kathleen joined us—"My girl," he said. Kathleen was a retired teacher and carefully researched everything she did. Doc had met her several years earlier, at a tag sale. He had seen cancer in her aura then, probably as a cloudy gray in her field, and suggested that she investigate it further. He also gave her his card, "something I never do." When she was diagnosed with breast cancer two years later, she made an appointment with him and they worked together to come up with a program to support her during the lumpectomy and radiation she had chosen. Before she met him, she knew nothing of alternative medicine. Now I know how difficult it had probably been for him to watch her go through the conventional medical treatment, which ran counter to everything he believed at that time. While Doc was full of conflict and erupting anger, Kathleen was utterly at peace with herself and the world. She glowed. She was one of the warmest human beings I have ever known. Sometimes I think she was sent to him toward the end as an angel of mercy.

Ten

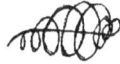

Doc, Again

November 1998-May 2001

"Your uterus is retroflexed and to the right," Doc said one day. I didn't know what I was supposed to do with that information. It wasn't giving me any trouble yet or, if it was, I had too many other things to worry about to notice.

Because he was very fond of Wilhelmina, my cat, Kathleen took Doc over to the Little Guild of St. Francis one day, and they returned with a gray cat he called Alley-Poo (Kathleen called her Alley Cat). Kathleen knew how much Doc needed companionship and, though he used to say he didn't like cats, he grew fond of Alley in spite of himself.

She outlived both of them.

Sometime after the lumpectomy and radiation, Kathleen's cancer recurred and was treated with Herceptin. This drug inhibits the HER-2 receptors on breast cancer cells. I am not certain, and wonder whether the medical establishment is certain, where else these receptors might be located and what effects inhibiting them in other locations might have. This was a new treatment at the time, and I don't think anyone was quite sure about how long it should be used. Doc put her on a number of heart-protective supplements that prevented the congestive heart failure that Herceptin can cause. I have heard of one person who was not so lucky, and I question the safety of a drug with this potentially fatal side effect. By taking Herceptin without adequate nutritional protection, are women going from the frying pan into the fire?

Kathleen had injections of Herceptin once a week for quite a long time, a year or two. The recurrence had started in a seemingly benign way, with a contact dermatitis on the arm that had the lymphedema. Lymphedema is a swelling of a limb resulting from poor lymphatic drainage, which can be the result of surgical removal of—or radiation damage to—lymph nodes. It is most commonly a side effect of surgical or radiation treatment of breast, prostate, uterine, or colon cancers. Kathleen's lymphedema didn't clear up as it should have, and she had had an ongoing problem with it. I used to treat it and had some success in bringing it down before the recurrence. A massage therapist in Maine treated it while Kathleen was there in the summer, and a clinic in Bangor gave her a hydraulic machine that pushed the fluid from the arm back toward the thorax.

The trouble with this, I think, was that too much of the lymphatics had been damaged by the combination of radiation and surgery, and when the fluid got back into the thorax, there was nowhere for it to go. My opinion is that a major factor in the development of breast cancer is inadequate lymphatic drainage, perhaps exacerbated by binding clothing (particularly bras), and also, perhaps, by the tendency of women to apply deodorants containing aluminum—where? Right in the armpit, which is full of lymph nodes, which are close to the surface and can easily absorb the ingredients through the skin. When Kathleen's cancer started growing again, it was right where the nodes to the arm were supposed to be draining into the thorax.

The power of castor oil packs

If I had to do it over again, I would strongly recommend that Kathleen do the Edgar Cayce castor oil packs (which, for some reason, Doc did not suggest). Gerson stated that cancer begins with the liver and the digestion. Castor oil packs, as described in the Cayce literature, are wool flannel cloths saturated with castor oil, most commonly applied over the liver for the systemic effect, although they can also be used topically. The castor oil is absorbed through the skin and stimulates the liver to do its detoxification work and hormone breakdown more efficiently. The packs also improve lymphatic flow and decrease bowel transit time, so that pathogens have less time to brew in the gut and cause leaky gut problems that could, in turn, become allergies and arthritis, due to foreign proteins getting into the blood that don't belong there. Pharmacologist and herbalist Earl Mindell, in *Earl Mindell's Herb Bible,* states that castor oil is one of more than seven hundred plant medicines mentioned in the Ebers Papyrus, written in Egypt around 1600 B.C. A former patient from Kenya told me that, in her native country, castor oil is used for bellyaches.

Cayce's prescriptions were always for individuals, not generic, so there are many different ways of using packs described in the readings, with or without heat, with varying frequencies, though Cayce often recommended three days on, four days off. My observation has been that the more toxic the patient's system is at the outset, the more cautious one has to be in the application of packs in order to avoid severe detoxification reactions.

My life out of balance

If Kathleen had used packs, the outcome might have been quite different, but I had a problem as a practitioner at this time. I was so busy that I had no time to research or think about things, only able to react to whatever crisis presented itself in the moment. My life was seriously out of balance and getting worse, as Doc, my mother, and the Workers' Comp patient were all getting sicker. Taking care of any one of them would have been a full-time job. I was falling behind all the time. My income did not reflect the amount of work I was doing, and this is when I began thinking that the practice was bleeding me to death.

It was, and my body heard me.

In the spring of 2000, I went to a Chinese restaurant for dinner. I had scallops and felt terrific! From this I drew the conclusion that I was short of iodine and started eating seaweed in my scrambled eggs every morning, a practice I continue to this day. So when I began light bleeding in September, I wasn't overly concerned, since I figured I was correcting a longstanding thyroid imbalance. The reason I came to this conclusion is that I once treated a patient who had had an injury to the thyroid. She told me that she had had no menstrual periods for the preceding six months, and her periods recommenced shortly after I began adjusting her neck.

In fact, I was correcting my own thyroid imbalance—but the imbalance was longer-standing than I thought. Doc was concerned and suggested I go to a gynecologist. I didn't have the time for that, and anyway, I didn't have anyone I felt comfortable working with at the time. "How can you be bleeding and still keep up your strength?" he asked me. One reason is the difference between men and women—as women, we are designed to lose a certain amount of blood every month. I do think, however, that I overdid it a bit. Another reason that I could continue to work under these conditions is that I was relatively young and strong.

Approaching exhaustion

Spring 2000 brought with it the opportunity to buy the house. This time, I was able to make an offer with the assurance that I would be able to carry the expense. The practice was continuing to build, as I kept creating more money for all the expenses that go into buying a house. Doc was beginning to lose ground. We were more concerned with the number of fender benders my mother was having. I remember going camping in Macedonia State Park during the summer, lying in the sleeping bag, listening to the brook. Then, for a split second, I didn't hear it, though I was conscious, and the brook had not stopped making brook sounds. I came to the insight that heart disease was an ultimate result and manifestation of exhaustion, and that was what I was coming to. I stopped hearing for a split second and can't explain why. I don't remember exactly how I pulled myself back from the brink that time, though I'm sure I couldn't have done it without the seaweed.

My life continued at the same speed and did not slow down, despite that warning. "You've got to learn to pace yourself," Doc said.

I had originally planned to close on the house in August, but the tenant wouldn't move out, so closing didn't happen until November. Jean did a tremendous amount of work cleaning, buying blinds and curtains, and making things ready so that I could move over from the old office as soon as possible. For slightly under two months I had the experience of walking to work, which I rather enjoyed.

I traditionally took the week between Christmas and New Year's off, so we planned the move for that week—some vacation! Toni came up from Yonkers with three movers, and I rented a fourteen-foot truck. Doc, Jean, Teresa, Shirley and I moved and organized pieces of furniture as they brought them in. Of course, there was snow on the ground (which there wouldn't have been in August). My birthday was a real gift from the universe—it was snowing so hard that we had the perfect excuse not to move any furniture. The view out the windows on the south side of the house was like a picture postcard, or the evergreens in the *Nutcracker* set. The Christmas lights on the house across the street were magical.

The Crew and I, Teresa, Jean, Shirley and Hummy, finished out the old year emptying out the old office and arranging the new office so that I could begin work again on Tuesday morning. Teresa sent me and Hummy to load out the old office while she and Shirley organized the new one. Toni had brought a rug for the reception room, which made it look much warmer and homier.

Whew! That was done. The ground was covered with snow until May that year. The tenant in the cottage had arranged for plowing, which was a Very Good Thing; as it was, we did a lot of shoveling anyway.

Doc and my practice take off

The practice took off like a rocket, while Doc was getting worse; I didn't realize quite how bad his condition was. Doc listened frequently to the news, with its usual collection of catastrophes and disasters, and would therefore become upset about whatever was going on at the moment. I learned from his example that this was something I shouldn't do. He was worrying about the price of gas, saying it would go up to two dollars a gallon by summer.

Wrong on two counts:

The price of gas didn't go up to two dollars a gallon that year.

Doc didn't make it until summer.

In May he went into the hospital for some procedure or other. I did not realize the gravity of it. After all, the PSA was normal! It turned out, however, that the cancer had metastasized to the bladder from the prostate. The PSA would not indicate this, as it only relates to the integrity (or not) of the prostate capsule. They had missed the metastasis to the bladder—which could actually have been caused by the radiation. Doc had asked me to be his health care proxy, and I had agreed. I wonder if I could have prevented some of the pain at the end, and maybe some pointless procedures, if I had been more proactive.

He was moved from the hospital to the nursing home across the street. At lunchtime on May 15 I stopped in to see him; he asked if I could bring in a clock so he could know what time it was. I said I would come back after I was through with my last patient.

Before I could get there, Kathleen called and told me he was gone.

In those last days of his, Doc and I had agreed that we would communicate with each other when one of us passed. I used to get communications from him through two friends of mine whom he did not know. He also came to say goodbye to me in a dream. Another time I saw someone with hair like his in the street.

And when I rock and roll on the Anatomotor, an old automated rolling table I inherited from him, sometimes it is as though he is treating me.

Eleven

"Atypical glandular cells of undetermined significance"

January 2002

The bleeding, which had begun in September 2000, was occurring on a daily basis now, but was still not very bad. Despite Doc's concern, I had had too much to do, with the purchase of the house and the escalating crises with my mother, to think about it. After two- and-a-half years of working closely with Doc twice a week, I was suddenly without a practitioner when he died in May 2001. With his death I also lost a dear friend, brilliant mentor and wonderful support. I was probably more shaken by this loss than I realized--the practice was still in overdrive, so I worked through the whole thing.

The universe decided I needed a practitioner, and stepped in. One month after Doc died, Jenny, who was fresh out of acupuncture school, came in with a back problem and suggested that we barter, as she needed a chiropractor and I needed an acupuncturist. This has turned out to be of outstanding mutual benefit.

Having studied some acupuncture in chiropractic school, I knew that it worked. What I studied was the cookbook version, with only a cursory explanation of context. Although I certainly fell far short of being an expert acupuncturist, I had had quite a bit of success with it in the clinic. What I did not yet understand was acupuncture's wide range of effectiveness, as it is utilized within the system in which it was designed. In allopathic medicine, one hears mostly about acupuncture in terms of pain control. This is rather akin to saying chiropractic's usefulness is restricted to low back pain—it does not even begin to approach the complexity and efficacy of the modality.

Jenny brings me Chinese medicine

Jenny describes Oriental medicine as "based on an energetic model recognizing the vital energy in all living things, which they [Eastern practitioners] call Qi. Inserting very thin needles into specific points on the energy channels of the body restores balance and smooths the flow of Qi. Each channel or meridian is associated with a specific organ and physiologic system. An imbalance or blockage in the meridians can cause pain and illness." The acupuncture points have been demonstrated to be points of increased electrical conductivity (lowered resistance) along the channels, so it stands to reason that the insertion of *metal needles* would influence the flow of energy (electricity). Some acupuncture points are of known anatomical significance; for example, some are "motor points," where nerve enters a muscle, while the anatomical significance of others remains unknown. The channels do not necessarily mirror the nervous system or known physical structures. They are organized into yin and yang channels. Yang channels are on the back of the body, where the sun shines, if you are lying prone or are a quadruped. The channels correspond to yin and yang organs. In the midline of the body, there is the *du* ("governing vessel") channel going up the back and the *ren* ("conception vessel") channel in the front.

The goal of acupuncture is to restore the smooth and unimpeded flow of Qi. Jenny describes cancer, "no matter where it is in the body, [as] an energetic and physiological imbalance….Acupuncture and Chinese Herbs rebalance the body, strengthen the immune system, address physical issues, and support the mental and emotional challenges of cancer." Jenny arrives at a treatment plan after careful questioning, examining the tongue for color, dampness or dryness, presence or absence and color of coating, and taking deep, middle, and superficial pulses at three points on each wrist.

Chinese medicine seems to have excellent success dealing with constitutional and hormonal issues with a consideration for the individual that Western medicine misses by a mile. After all, Western medicine is only now beginning to acknowledge the subtle energies that the Chinese have been studying in depth for five thousand years or so. Western medicine is more accurate with regard to anatomy and structure, and still knows practically nothing of the energies that animate the structure.

Jenny is a Reiki Master as well as an acupuncturist. She determined at the beginning that I was not protecting my energy adequately and absorbing too much from the patients. She mentioned specifically a "vortex at the third chakra." I had never been formally taught my method of working; it had developed over a period of many years and, consequently, I also had not learned any methods of energy protection. The need for and methods of energy protection are not taught in chiropractic school. (I have been told that they are not taught in seminary, either.) In ignoring the very real existence of energy and the problems thereof—since the subject is considered scientifically unproven— these and other institutions are doing a grave disservice to their graduates, subjecting them to the increased likelihood of stress and mental or physical illness. Massage therapists and energy workers are in the vanguard in the self-protection arena, and "mainstream" professionals would do well to learn from them.

Jenny taught me some techniques for energy protection. She said that other people's energy comes in at the solar plexus (Caroline Myss says so, too). Therefore she suggested wearing orange over the solar plexus when I work. I found a huge improvement in my energy when I started doing this. She also suggested spraying the treatment room with a spray made with local spring water and sage and eucalyptus essential oils to clear the energy in the room. She, Jean, and Teresa can all feel the thickness in the energy more than I can, and will often tell me that I need to spray the room, since I sometimes forget. If I, myself, can tell that the energy in the room is thick, it must be pretty bad! I also sometimes wear bracelets that help prevent my absorbing the patients' energy electrically. This is particularly important for me, as I work by letting the impulses from their nervous systems run through mine, and use my nervous system to read theirs.

Jenny and I tried for the next six months to stop the bleeding. Nothing worked. She suggested I get it checked out.

"Atypical glandular cells"

So, in 2002, after the Christmas holidays, I made an appointment at the local clinic with a nurse practitioner who had been recommended to me. The Pap came out with the highly equivocal "atypical" result shown above. "Glandular" cells means that the questionable cells are from the uterus and not the cervix. I was thinking I might have become anemic, due to the bleeding, but money was still short after the move, so the nurse practitioner did a finger stick instead of a complete blood count and found that my hemoglobin was 14, which is about where it usually was. So I wasn't anemic yet.

The nurse practitioner said that the next diagnostic step would be either an ultrasound or an endometrial biopsy. An ultrasound would show if there were abnormal thickening of the endometrium. A biopsy, considered the "gold standard," would show aberrations in individual cell structure, but not necessarily the extent of the problem. I said I was not willing to have a hysterectomy, in any case.

"What if it will save your life?" she asked. "I don't think it will," I said to myself. Then she asked what I considered to be a very bizarre question under the circumstances: "Are you concerned about osteoporosis?" I said no, which effectively ended that conversation, as I wondered to myself why she was trying to sell me a DEXA scan when we were thinking about a possible cancer. Those considered to be most at risk for osteoporosis are thin white women who smoke. I am a woman and I am white, but I am not thin and have never smoked, and furthermore have been physically active most of my life. There is a continuum of estrogen balance; on the low-estrogen side is the risk of osteoporosis, whereas on the high-estrogen side is the risk of endometrial cancer. It was quite clear to me where I was on that continuum. To figure that out, all I had to do was look in the mirror.

She referred me to a local gynecologist, a male. I don't see male gynecologists, so didn't make an appointment, though several women have spoken well of him.

Jenny asked if I had tried castor oil packs, one of the most frequently recommended remedies in the Edgar Cayce material. I said I'd thought about doing them. "What about now?" she asked. I did the first one that night.

Twelve

Retest: More of the Same

March 2002

After two months of castor oil packs, I set up an appointment with Dr. Abby, a gynecologist who was highly recommended to me. She had moved further west in the area, which is why it had not occurred to me to go to her earlier. The bleeding was increasing somewhat, but in general I was feeling considerably better, due to the castor oil packs. My uterus, which had had a boggy feel at the time I began the packs, had considerably improved in tone. I knew this intuitively, and also by the way it felt when I was adjusting her (my uterus), using my own approach, combining chiropractic and acupressure. I also noted that the yeast infection I had in January was gone, and that a fungus toenail I had had for several years had cleared up, all due to the castor oil packs. I had decided that I would retest after resolving the yeast infection to see if it made any difference.

It didn't.

Dr. Abby and I discussed the next step; she recommended an endometrial biopsy. I was uninsured at this point and figured I had a choice between the biopsy and a much-needed vacation. I chose the vacation.

The American Cancer Society wouldn't agree with me, but it was the right thing to do.

I had decided to go to Virginia Beach to investigate the A.R.E., Edgar Cayce's Association for Research and Enlightenment, since I had never been there. Tonia had told me about taking a vacation in Virginia Beach with her father and her daughter, and had described Cape May and the ferry between Cape May and Lewes. It sounded delightful to me—I love ferryboats and was also looking forward to seeing the Victorian houses at Cape May. So I left at 9:00 p.m. in a pelting rainstorm.

The flooding began somewhere on either the Jersey Turnpike or the Garden State. I am referring to extremely heavy bleeding, not to the roads. I stopped for the night somewhere in South Jersey, walked around Cape May in the morning, and then took the ferry to Lewes in the early afternoon. I was heading south from there when I noticed that the car's fan belt was acting up again, so I drove back to Lewes, where there was a Jeep dealer. I found a motel within walking distance and dropped the Jeep off at the dealer's, where it remained for three days.

Could I possibly have received a clearer message that I needed to slow down and be fully present where I was?

When I was not flooding, which tended to be worse in the evening, I explored Lewes on foot. Lewes has a museum, the Zwaanendael (Valley of the Swans) museum, which tells the story of a small band of Dutch settlers who landed there in the 1600s. The museum is modeled after the city hall of Hoorn, in Holland, where the settlers came from. Unfortunately, they came to a bad end.

The flooding was getting quite intense; I was passing a number of large clots. It was not consistent but would wane and then begin again suddenly. I didn't feel any particular weakness, simply relief after the current bout was over. Finally, the Jeep was ready, and Sarah, the owner of the motel, gave me a ride over to the dealer's to pick it up. And I hit the road. She told me it was about four hours to Virginia Beach, so I decided to go for it.

On the drive down, the flooding intensified again, requiring me to make several stops along the way. It was getting so bad that I had to stop for the night, which turned out to be at the Rittenhouse Motel in Cape Charles, Virginia. It was a beautiful place, attentively landscaped by Mr. Rittenhouse over the last fifty years.

The flooding was still increasing. I was up and down all night; I would no sooner lie down than it would start up again. Up and down, up and down. Finally, toward morning, I decided to stand in the shower and let it do whatever it wanted.

The body in control after all

After a while, it stopped.

This showed me that my body was in control of the process and would not let the bleeding go on beyond what was safe. Endometrial cancer is often initially diagnosed by ultrasound, and is suspected if the endometrial stripe is wider than 5mm. This means that the endometrium is thicker than it ought to be. Flooding is the body's natural way to thin it out. I knew, from that time on, that I would not end up hemorrhaging in the hospital, because the bleeding had a purpose and would stop when that purpose was fulfilled.

In the morning I took the Chesapeake Bay Bridge-Tunnel to Virginia Beach. The first order of business was to find a laundromat. By this time I didn't have a lot of my vacation left, so after some walking on the beach, a tour of the A.R.E. and some exploration of the Heritage Store, it was time to go home again. I picked up a brochure from the A.R.E. Health Center describing their half-day spa packages. I was considering the possible benefits of colonics for Jean and Teresa as well as for myself.

The flooding was never quite that bad again. It continued on an intermittent basis, though some bleeding was a daily occurrence. Initially it seemed to have some vague relationship to a menstrual cycle. Was I going through the change? Maybe. Maybe not. At 53, it could have been either way. In one sense, I don't know what menopause is, because I've never had it. In another way, I've experienced the change in overdrive, even choosing some herbs by referring to Susun Weed's *The Menopausal Years.* The cancer has behaved a great deal like the menopause I didn't have.

I found that working too hard brought on flooding. I found that the gong meditation in yoga class brought on flooding. I also found that I usually felt better after flooding than before. It might be an exaggeration to say that I felt well, but I had an absolute certainty that my body was doing what it needed to. So I figured I would retest in the fall—that would be time enough.

Thirteen

Lyme Disease

S o after a few months of flooding, on and off, it came to be summer, and I went camping over July 4 weekend with friends. It was extremely hot, the brush was overgrown, and everything was biting. I had just had the cottage roof replaced to the tune of $4000, so savings were low. The practice was still going full throttle until July 16, when I found it becoming more and more of a struggle to keep going as the day wore on.

Toward the end of the day I was spiking a fever and had shooting pains down both legs. I asked Teresa to call and cancel all the patients, and went to bed, drinking gallons of water and taking Vitamin C lozenges non-stop. One of the patients—a new one—didn't get the message and showed up the next day for her adjustment. I did well and have the notes to prove it and don't remember a thing.

After nearly a week of nonstop Vitamin C, rolling on the Ana-tomotor (Doc's automatic rolling table) two to four times a day, and daily castor oil packs, I still was eating nothing but canned fruit, and the fever was persisting at 101.5. I thought maybe I ought to go to check for tick bites in the upstairs mirror, but didn't even have the energy to do that. So I didn't argue with Teresa when she suggested I go to the MDs and have it checked out. It was Lyme disease, which I had thought was a distinct possibility. Lyme disease and ehrlichiosis are both endemic in Dutchess County, where I live. They put me on doxycycline for a month.

By 4 a.m. the fever had started to drop. Bloodwork showed cholesterol at 149, liver enzymes elevated, and anemia. During the bout of Lyme disease, I didn't bleed very much. In addition to the doxycycline, I used whatever I had in the way of supplements and herbs that applied to the situation. Symptoms were mostly neurological—after the fever broke, and with the aid of castor oil packs and herbal supports, I had relatively little in the way of muscle and joint pains or headache. I couldn't read the micro-wave clock from across the room, however, and mentally I had moments of crystal brilliance alternating with not having a clue. My energy was erratic. In yoga class, I couldn't do the exercises involving turning my head without getting dizzy.

For two weeks I didn't work at all. Then the following week I treated one patient per day. Then I increased to seeing two patients per day, then three, with naps in between. I came off the doxycycline in one month, as planned. This seemed to be enough. I was more than willing to give up the gassiness caused by the antibiotic and also found that it caused a certain amount of stiffness and dehydration. The Lyme didn't rebound after I stopped the doxycycline. The visual symptoms were the slowest to go away, and especially if I was driving late at night, one eye would get very sore. The fatigue persisted for some time. In fact, I wondered if I would ever have the energy to walk up the hill again. The bloodwork still showed anemia, though the liver enzymes had normalized, so I started on Herbal Iron. Jenny also added some Chinese herbs and used shi shen gong, a needle pattern at the crown of the head and cupping the back, which was very helpful for the stiffness. The effect of shi shen gong was very similar to what I can do with cranial adjusting.

My energy was slow in returning as I gradually increased the patient load to four per day. But by September I was still not in any frame of mind to pursue diagnostic issues any further (having had quite enough of doctors), so I didn't. I was mostly focused on trying to get some energy back. By late August I was able to walk about two miles again. Money was short after a summer of much decreased work load, so as winter approached I was attempting to push up to seven patients a day again. This was a mistake, and I found that I could not do it.

The upside of Lyme

The Lyme disease, in a strange way, represented a brief return to a sort of sanity, as during that period I was only doing what I could handle. I was even able to write a little bit—a piece called *Fun with Lyme,* an account of my dealing with the Lyme, how it felt and what I did for it as it happened, containing a lot of detail I would have otherwise forgotten. I still use this as a patient information piece on Lyme. I felt a sort of normalcy in the fall, since I felt so much better than I had with Lyme—it was almost like being healthy.

But the family was pressuring me, so I told them I planned to have a diagnosis for them by Christmas. I reflected on what kind of an answer that should be—I had originally thought I would repeat the Pap again, but that would have been a waste of time, as it would merely have said the same thing without providing a real answer.

And did I really want a diagnosis anyway? I was—and am—all too familiar with the negative effects a diagnosis can have: People have been known to lose hope and die on the basis of a diagnosis, correct or not. Was it going to change what I was going to do? I had decided that I did not want a hysterectomy. I asked myself, what did I really fear most about cancer? I knew that there is a lot of negativity connected with a cancer diagnosis, and it regularly assumes almost mythic proportions. Somehow cancer has come to be set apart from other conditions by Western medicine, provoking an all-out assault on the patient by the very doctors who are supposed to be helping. Conventional Western cancer therapy is, by nature, cruel and violent—and, in my opinion, has a problem coming to the right conclusion because it starts from the wrong premise.

Healthy fear of the medical industry

What I feared most about the cancer, then, was not the cancer itself, but the prospect of losing control over my own body and my own destiny and handing it over to the tender mercies of doctors and hospitals, with the possibility of error compounded upon error keeping me married to doctors and hospitals, which I don't like. I also suspected that none of this was necessary, as I trusted my body to know what she was doing.

What was my chief problem, as I saw it? Exhaustion. What is the cure for exhaustion? I didn't think it was major surgery.

This being the case, I decided in the end to go for the biopsy and get a diagnosis. This put me under no obligation whatsoever to accept the conventional treatment. I would simply skip it. I had handled the Lyme disease well, using mostly what I had available in the kitchen. I trusted my skills more than I had the year before. Putting off the diagnosis had not been a conscious decision, but was the hidden wisdom of the universe, which in this instance served me well. I would not have had the confidence to attempt treating a cancer myself before having the experience of working with Lyme. If Western medicine had had some equivalent of a month of doxycycline to offer in the way of cancer treatment, I might have considered it.

Fourteen

"Endometrioid Adenocarcinoma"

December 20, 2002

It was ten days before my 54th birthday. The Crew and I were scheduled to gather for our traditional holiday dinner at the Round Tuit after my gynecological appointment that would give me the result of the biopsy. Sandra, who had been through something similar herself many years before, came to the doctor's office to support me.

"It's cancer," Dr. Abby said. "The conventional way of dealing with it is hysterectomy."

Being in the business, I had some idea of the risks of hysterectomy—not only the risks of infection, hemorrhage, or nerve damage that are always inherent in major surgery, but I also knew that my hormone balance would never be right again. I had considered this issue and frankly preferred to take my chances dealing with the cancer my way. "No slashing, burning, or poisoning," I told the gynecologist.

"It [hysterectomy] can be devastating," she agreed. *(I wondered, would she have said that if I had chosen a hysterectomy?)*

She said she was concerned and referred me to a local osteopath for nutritional help, though I decided later that Jenny and I could handle that aspect ourselves. Dr. Abby asked that I write every couple of months and let her know how things were going.

After we left the doctor's office, as I remember it, Sandra and I drove to the Round Tuit to join The Crew. During the drive, she told me that her mother had had a hysterectomy for a precancerous condition. "Before, she was an aging woman. After, she was an aged woman." My friends were waiting to hear the diagnosis, and my report cast a pall over the evening. Jean gave me her reindeer antler headband. "I think you need this."

Sandra recalls this day somewhat differently and tells me that she and I had supper alone at Four Brothers. We discussed how I was going to handle it, and this is where I came up with the idea of writing the letter to the family. Why is this important? It shows me that I was more upset than I remember, to the extent of affecting my recall of the events of that day.

The elephant in the dining room

I was dreading Christmas dinner with my family. My mother had been over at Stamford Hospital, having a series of radiation treatments for a brain tumor, and was going to be let out for the day to join us, so I decided to say nothing about the diagnosis, but rather to hand everyone a letter afterward, in which I made it clear what I was planning to do, and in which I asked that they keep any misgivings they might have to themselves. My sister Fran, her husband, Michael, son Mikie and father-in-law Arthur were there, as well as my sister Janet, our close friends Toni and Frank, and my mother. During the whole evening I was most aware of the elephant in the living room and I suspect everyone else was, too. There was a heavy snowstorm, and I followed Janet's car in mine when we left. There was no way I could make it the rest of the way home, so I stayed with her that night and handed her the letter. She read it and said that it was up to me, since she didn't know anything about these matters.

It had not really occurred to me that the family might be opposed to or have concerns about the way I was handling the cancer. I was looking at my situation from the viewpoint of having been in practice for almost eight years and having formed some definite opinions about healing in general and healing cancer in particular.

I felt that the conventional medical paradigm was starting from an incorrect premise, which would therefore make it difficult to come to the correct conclusion. I saw (and still see) no point in working hard to kill the cancer only to destroy the body's energy and vitality in the process. If, for example, my energy level were at 80% at the time of diagnosis, surgery would bring it down to 50%, even barring complications. I would then find it much harder to get back up to the original 80% than if I had not had surgery at all.

Why not work directly from 80% and try to go higher?

The allopathic trap

My observation has been that, once one starts down the garden path of allopathic medicine—with surgery, drugs, or whatever—it becomes increasingly difficult to get off it, as complications can beget complications. Surgery, like courtroom justice, is always a wild card. To my mind, the risks of undergoing a hysterectomy were far greater than the risks presented by the cancer itself. I had already lived with the bleeding for over two years. It was not progressing rapidly, it was not fulminating—raging out of control—so I was not hemorrhaging uncontrollably. I figured I had time.

My general health was actually better than it had been a couple of years before. I had handled the recent bout with Lyme disease well, considering that I had been living with an undiagnosed cancer at the time, simply by taking the month's worth of doxycycline and whatever other herbs and supplements I had on hand that I felt applied to the situation. The Crew and other friends in Amenia respected both my decision and my ability to make it. What I realized later was that my family did not recognize me as a doctor, and therefore it was much harder for them to trust that I knew what I was doing.

My sisters, Mimi, Janet, and Fran, kept their concerns to themselves, as I had asked, but other dear friends found it hard to accept my decision and tried to change my mind in various ways. Jean and Teresa served a vital function by running interference for me.

So what tack was I going to take to treat the cancer? (Susun Weed: *Step 1: Gather information.*) Upon Jean's and Sharon's suggestion, I met with Mike and Maureen, who are Hare Krishnas, at Calsi's General Store. They shared their experience with the Gerson therapy in the 1970s. As vegetarians, they objected to Gerson's use of liver juice and substituted a combination of beet juice and whey protein. They also talked about the herbal work of Dr. John Christopher. They lent me their copy of Dr. Gerson's book, *A Cancer Therapy: Results of Fifty Cases,* and *My Triumph over Cancer,* by Beata Bishop, who had recovered from metastasized melanoma using the Gerson Therapy. Beata Bishop's book was important to me because it gave me valuable insights into the healing process and, in particular, what I might expect from detoxification as well as the usefulness of taking it slowly in order to avoid the "flare-ups," healing crises that plagued her at various points in her healing process and are an expected aspect of the Gerson Therapy.

I decided I wasn't sick enough to need to do full-scale Gerson, though I knew I needed to add something to my present protocol. If one is doing Gerson, at least in the early stages, one does nothing else. I was still working my practice and expected to continue to work, so whatever therapies I chose had to be possible in that context. As a Blood Type O, macrobiotics did not appeal to me. I needed meat. This had become clear to me during my recovery from Lyme. I knew I wasn't willing to put that kind of effort and energy into the cooking that macrobiotics requires, and anyway, I didn't feel it would meet my protein and iron needs sufficiently to compensate for the flooding, the intermittent, but at times severe bleeding. I did know that I was exhausted, and that my trying to return to a full work schedule (seven patients per day, spending an hour apiece on average) after the Lyme disease had been a serious mistake. I decided to cut down to no more than five patients per day.

A gift from the Ojibway is under attack

The next time I saw Jenny for acupuncture, she added Essiac to the protocol. Many attempts to introduce it to Western medicine had always been stonewalled by the medical establishment. We tried the Resperin version (Resperin owns the rights to the name Essiac) and FlorEssence before eventually settling on Four + One, the version sold by Jean's Greens, which was much less expensive and equally effective. Upon Joy's suggestion, I also added fresh carrot, apple and lemon juice, one 16-ounce glass daily, to the protocol.

I was on this formula for about five years and never suffered any ill effects from it. Not only was it useful in coping with the cancer; it also helped me handle sugar better, and indeed these two properties may be related. It seems to help one's system run cleaner, from what I have observed. This doesn't sound controversial, does it?

Apparently, it is. I was talking with Holly, the current owner of Jean's Greens, and she told me that Jean, the original owner, had made some flyers about her version of Essiac that mentioned the word "cancer." Oops! The FDA saw them and gave her a warning to remove all mention of cancer from her flyers. She did so but apparently missed some. So the FDA, the guardians of our health, who haven't been able to protect us from that antibiotic that ruptures tendons, nor the radiation and chemo that cause new cancers to develop after "treating" the old ones, nor from the Herceptin that can cause congestive heart failure, raided her store and seized her entire supply of the herbal formula and its components. Apparently she decided to sell the business, due to FDA harassment.

Centuries of success not "evidence-based"

Manufacturers of herbs and supplements are not allowed to claim any effectiveness for their products in diagnosing or treating any disease, even if there are studies to prove their effectiveness or hundreds or thousands of years of tradition, as in the case of some Western and Chinese herbs. The result of this is that the FDA, far from protecting the right of the people to treat their diseases as they see fit, is keeping potentially life-saving information from them and raiding herbalists and supplement manufacturers, while letting the pharmaceutical industry do exactly as it pleases.

Thus, with the addition of Essiac, what became my basic protocol for most conditions was in place. Jenny altered the Chinese herbs to include Red Flower, to prevent metastasis, Zedo Compound to target the Essiac to the lower *dan tien* (the belly in Chinese medicine, lowest of three power centers), and Ba Zhen Wan to build the blood. The first week after starting the Essiac, I felt weak and feverish, as the herbs kicked my immune system into gear. Fortunately, this was the week between Christmas and New Year's and I wasn't working anyway.

Friends and community gathered round and offered incredible support. Joy offered to do fourteen sessions of Guided Imagery and Music with me, to help assess and get to the root of the problem, and to find out what the body was saying about it. And I decided that—never mind whether I could afford it or not—Tonia and I would drive down to Florida to visit Tevie and Jano and make a stop in Virginia Beach, headquarters of Edgar Cayce's A.R.E., along the way. Never having had a colonic in fifty-four years, and figuring that the major components of the healing process were to be detoxification and rebuilding, I scheduled the half-day spa package at the A.R.E.—castor oil pack, manual lymphatic drainage, acupressure, and colonic.

Fifteen

Shamanic Journey

January 2003

I was busy at home in early January.

There I was with a diagnosis, like it or not. As it turned out, having a diagnosis was tremendously important. It did change what I was going to do. I recognized it as an imperative to do what the body wanted *right then* and not fool around any more.

I resigned from active care of my mother in the infamous Christmas letter I wrote to my family. The diagnosis had made it possible for me to say no. I hope that the next time I have to say no I won't have to get cancer in order to do it.

I also dispensed promptly with any inclination to ramp up my practice again.

Jean, Joy, and Dr. Fran from Chicago plied me with a number of useful books and, following Susun Weed's first step (*Gather Information),* I read and reread pieces of them, not in any particular order, but as seemed germane to the issue at hand. Dr. Fran had sent me a letter with tips from a member of her Reiki circle who had been working on healing breast cancer that had metastasized to bone. Also in the letter was a sheet describing the Emotional Freedom Technique, which I used effectively later on.

EFT is a branch of energy medicine based on the science of Kinesiology. It's a way of resolving emotional issues quickly, often providing instant relief by clearing the energy meridians through a simple tapping technique. EFT is easy to learn and infinitely relevant to our lives. Free information about EFT is available online.

It was also during this time that I sat down at the computer and compiled a list of all the factors I could think of that could contribute to cancer. After countless revisions, this has evolved into *Toward an Individualized Treatment of Cancer,* which is now a chapter in this book. I designed it as a decision tree to be used in weighing the appropriateness of different therapies, according to the strengths and weaknesses of the person using them. For instance, someone with a cancer diagnosis and a severe toxicity problem—such as someone who smokes, drinks, uses medical or recreational drugs, eats badly, or works with toxic chemicals—would be most likely to benefit from the rigorous discipline of the Gerson Therapy, whereas I did not feel it was necessary for me.

Guided imagery and music: good therapy

Joy generously offered a therapy that I found extremely helpful and enlightening. She is a musician and music therapist who also holds a Master's degree in Special Education, and was a Special Ed teacher at a local school at that time. She is also a Reiki Master, because her instructor in the Helen Bonny method of Guided Imagery and Music told her that it is vitally important to be conversant with some kind of energy work when doing this type of therapy. Joy had taken the two-year GIM training in Virginia Beach and had become familiar with the Edgar Cayce work at that time. She, who was to be a tremendous help and support over the next six months, described to me the Helen Bonny method of Guided Imagery and Music: "It can help you cut through to the essentials much more quickly than talk therapy," she said. "Usually we use a series of either seven or fourteen sessions. At the beginning of each one, we talk about what you want to work on that day. Then I play a selection of music and you talk about whatever it brings up. At the end of the session, you draw a mandala, give it a title, and initial and date it."

Before the sessions began, she would administer the MARI test, which she said was designed by an art therapist. According to www.musicinhealth.net, "The MARI [Mandala Assessment Research Institute] card test is a non-verbal way of gaining insight into one's present state—in mind, body and spirit. Art therapist Joan Kellogg developed this method in 1978, based upon art therapy principles, consciousness research, Jungian theory and cross-cultural studies. Amazingly simple, the card test provides insights difficult to find through words."

I would be shown a number of shapes and colors, pick the ones I liked the most and the least, and match colors to the shapes. She said that we would repeat the test at the end of the sessions, but we never got around to that. One of the shapes I chose indicated the presence of new growth—the cancer.

Joy and I got off to a rip-roaring start just after New Year's. During the first session I went promptly to my funeral in a military past life. I was above, looking down. I had been good at what I did, and successful in the military sense, but I suspected I hadn't been very nice. I made a comment to Joy on the fact that war does not work as a method of solving problems. Then I felt myself slammed into another incarnation as a sickly child in some cold climate, I believe in the British Isles somewhere. It was quite abrupt. I was having trouble breathing. "Can you call for help?" Joy asked.

"I can't. I'm being strangled." I was in some culture where that was how they dealt with crippled children. "It was the adult males who did it."

About a month before that, I had seen the movie *The Talented Mr. Ripley*. In the final scene, Tom Ripley strangles his lover, whose back is turned because he trusts him. I had found it extremely upsetting, and I usually don't react to movies that way.

The necessary practice of receiving

My mother used to say that I had been afraid of strange places when I was a baby, so when we went to visit my grandmother she would leave me in the car, where I would fall asleep. She would explain, "That's just the way she is." I am fairly sure that it relates somehow back to that lifetime of being strangled, and I am also fairly sure that it had nothing to do with my mother or any of the current cast of characters. What an act of courage it is to be a parent, with children coming into life carrying a collection of fears and neuroses for which you are probably not responsible, and which you know nothing about.

Joy commented in the early sessions that it was difficult to get me to stay with and in my body. It is much easier now; I can tune into my body at will and have often used this facility to communicate with my uterus. (More on that later.) I give the GIM sessions with Joy credit for that facility, which has been necessary in the healing process. During the first session I was complaining because here I was doing healing work, which I felt was my purpose in life and what I had been called to do, and had nevertheless come down with cancer. Joy had no answer for this, but did ask, "Are you supposed to be working now?"

"No," I said.

This being a definite answer, I decided to stop worrying about whether I could afford to travel down to Florida with Tonia, and just go. After all, what better opportunity would we have? We would be delivering Jano's car to her, so would only have to drive in one direction. If being diagnosed with cancer wasn't an important enough reason to go on vacation, I couldn't think of a better one. It also seemed to me a pretty clear choice: life vs. anti-life.

Healing prayer figured importantly in those early days. Shortly after I was diagnosed, Joy and I went to a healing service at the Oratory of the Little Way in Gaylordsville, Connecticut, which was held, coincidentally, on our mutual birthday. The next week Rev. Carl, the pastor of the Sharon Methodist Church, came over to my house with Jean and Teresa to pray with me.

Dona and Tonia called a healing circle for me before Tonia and I left for Virginia Beach and Florida. I spoke first, then we went around the circle and everyone spoke. I remember more of the power of the vibrations and the strength of the support than the specifics, and for many months afterward I would feel that force once again whenever we sang the "Ra, ma, da, sa, sa, say, so hung" ("Sun, moon, earth, ether, I am that balance or infinity") mantra in yoga class. I do remember lying on the table during the circle and receiving, as everyone came around and offered his or her own unique style of prayers and blessings. As would prove to be true again, sound and vibration were integral to this circle.

Another clairvoyant sees the problem

Tonia and I went to Virginia Beach on the way to Florida. I had little chance to explore there the previous March. I planned to include the Lymph Cleanse this trip and make it an integral part of my detoxification program twice a year. Playing in the bookstores wouldn't hurt, either. Traveling with Tonia was always a guaranteed adventure, as she would strike up conversation with just about anybody, and I could just follow along for the ride and not have to say much of anything. It was jolly good fun. Each morning we would draw a card from the Tarot of the Spirit deck to set the tone for the day. Mine always seemed to be about transformation and life-changing events. On this trip we established what would become our Virginia Beach rituals—carrot juice and lunch at the Heritage Cafe, book shopping at the Heritage and the A.R.E., the Lymph Cleanse, a hot tub room overlooking the ocean at the Schooner. It was bitter cold and windy in January, and one day, as the wind was howling and a couple of inches of snow were falling, we were interviewed in the Heritage Store because we had braved the weather. Of course, the snow was nothing in comparison to what we had left behind, and, when we returned home, everyone told us about the sub-zero temperatures they had weathered.

We were loath to leave Virginia Beach because we were having such a good time, but, thinking that Jano might want her car sometime, we decided to set off on Friday morning. Tonia thought it might be fun if we made an appointment to see a psychic. This is how we met Belinda.

She took my left hand. "You have a health problem," she said. "What is it?" I told her I had just been diagnosed with endometrial cancer. "You can beat this thing," she said. "Uterus is the mother." Either I told her or she picked up psychically that I was worried about finances, and she reassured me that I wouldn't lose the house. At this point I had absolutely no clue as to how sick I might get. "I see a lot of activity going on," she said, "construction." She saw the front porch being repaired, but couldn't tell if a ramp was being added or not (something I had been considering since I bought the house, but I couldn't seem to come up with a design solution I liked). It was still quite soon after my mother's series of radiation treatments and I didn't know yet how far they were going to take her down, so I asked Belinda about caring for my mother, though on another level I was certain I could not do it. She told me she was directed to give me a small silver pendulum, which I use from time to time to assess my energy and to check foods and vitamins to see whether I should be taking them at the moment.

We drove on to Florida. Everywhere along the way people were complaining about the unseasonable cold. We stopped at Pedro's South of the Border and bought a flamingo hat to bring to Tevie. The weather remained cold until we woke up in Jacksonville; then we were finally able to bring out the Florida clothes we had bought along the way.

After spending a few peaceful days with Jano and her daughter Tevie (who looked stunning in the flamingo hat), sightseeing, walking on the beach, and dining out, we went into Sarasota to meet Judith, who had recently moved there from a small town near Albany. She had a number of activities planned; the following morning, we set out bright and early for Warm Mineral Springs an hour or so south of Sarasota. Like a number of other places in Florida, this claims to be the actual Fountain of Youth searched for and missed by Ponce de Leon. Whether or not it was, it was delightful. There was a pool (natural, not artificial) with trees around it; the center, from which the spring water welled up, was two hundred feet deep. It had a decidedly Eastern European flavor. Doc would have been at home there, and would definitely have approved, having often recommended that I go to hot springs or a hot tub. Elderly ladies and gentlemen bobbed in the water wearing sun hats and sunglasses. Pierogies were served at the snack bar. We talked to a woman who was sitting in the water plastering green mud on her face. "Don't tell anyone," she said, "I don't think I'm supposed to." We also met a young man with MS who had been staying at the nearby cottages so that he could go to the springs every day.

A message from the uterus

I was pleasantly exhausted when we returned to Judith's that night, and I had a strong, emphatic and almost angry message from my uterus: "Your mother has to know." I would have to tell her about the cancer when I returned home. The chemistry of the mineral spring water made thoughts and sensations extraordinarily vivid, an effect I also noticed on a subsequent trip after sitting in the ocean water at Assateague Island off the Virginia coast.

Judith had recently joined the Unity Church in Sarasota. The pastors, Revs. Don and Dorothy Ann, were hosting a potluck for new members, and Judith invited us to go along with her. It was a large and friendly gathering of about forty warm and interesting people, each of whom spoke in turn and introduced themselves. We were the last in the circle. Tonia, who isn't shy about very much, told everyone that I had just been diagnosed with cancer and was not planning to treat it medically. Revs. Don and Dorothy Ann asked me to get in the middle of the circle, and they all sang my name.

Rev. Don, who looked hale and hearty, said he had been diagnosed with prostate cancer four years before and was treating it with homeopathic injections--the Homeopathic Activator of the Natural Immune System (HANSI) protocol developed by Argentinian biologist Juan Jose Hirschmann. HANSI International has headquarters in Sarasota.

We also attended a Native American powwow and a Scottish festival, and then returned home.

I had had an imperative from the body (the message from my uterus to tell my mother) and was not looking forward to following it. My oldest sister Mimi did not think I should tell my mother, and I had a letter from a close friend telling me she thought it would be a horrible thing to do. I did not agree.

Soon after our return, I went to see my mother in New Canaan. My sister Fran had flown east to be near our mother after her series of radiation treatments, and was very helpful in broaching the subject when it came to be time for me to tell her about the cancer. My mother said she would have been extremely hurt if she had not been told. I had known that.

Soon after I got back to Amenia, my mother called. Generally she had a very hard time hearing, understanding, or thinking clearly over the phone, so we didn't usually talk on the phone much. On this occasion, however, she was absolutely clear, understood and considered thoughtfully everything I said, and told me she loved me.

We hadn't had as clear a conversation as this one in at least two years.

Sixteen

Considering Dying

Spring 2003

Eventually—too soon—it was time to leave the warm mineral springs and helpful psychics and others who had made our odyssey unforgettable. After a mere two weeks away, in which so much had happened, it was time to go back to work. At home, I no longer slept on the second floor, where I could hear the telephone, but retreated to the much more peaceful space on the third floor. I looked at work differently now—in case of an emergency, I would consider, *are they in more trouble than I am?*

In many cases, they weren't.

I was juicing and taking Essiac on a daily basis. Jenny was treating me once a week. The practice, while scaled down, was still busy enough.

In February, the universe got to work again. The phone rang one afternoon. It was Dr. Heather, a young chiropractor who was a family friend of my mother's MD.

"I heard you might need some help," she said. We met soon thereafter and I found her likable and intelligent, and saw that her personal fitness training background would be an asset to the practice. She was located in Stamford, near my mother, so the first thing I had her do was take over my mother's care. Since the radiation treatments, my mother's energy had gone seriously downhill, and she was on seizure medication, which made her fall asleep at the table. Furthermore, after the radiation her skin was tight and painful, which it hadn't been before. Heather did well with my mother at first, though ultimately there wasn't a lot she could do, as things got worse.

Is this what dying is like?

I was getting more exhausted by the day and had to consider the possibility that the protocols I was using to treat the cancer might not work. Actually, it was too soon to tell. There were days when I could barely stir from the back porch and would wonder, *Is this what dying is like?* Then I figured it probably wasn't, because dying was what my mother was doing, and she couldn't walk, and couldn't feed herself, etc, etc....So I figured I still had quite a way to go. I read *The Tibetan Book of Living and Dying;* I read *When Things Fall Apart,* by Pema Chodron. The Tibetans were most helpful at this point, with their dispassionate discussions of bardo states, of the process of dying, and of groundlessness. I was in quite a state of groundlessness. The Tibetans speak of the value of rehearsing dying. In a sense, that's what I was doing. It wasn't the same as depression. It was closer to a state of neutral mind. I was just *being*, not having the energy to do much else.

Moira gave me some lily bulbs that spring, four of them. I knew they needed to go in the ground and wondered if I would ever have the energy to put them in. Every year, when they come up and bloom with their pink and white flowers, I am reminded of that time. And I take a moment for gratitude.

It was becoming clearer that I could heal myself, or I could work at my practice, but I could not do both. If I worked and didn't heal, ultimately I wouldn't be able to do either one, so I decided in May that I would take the month of June off. It would be diagnostics time in June again, and I always figure if I am good and do the diagnostics, I can reward myself by getting out of town. The insurance (later referred to as the "stupid insurance") had officially kicked in in January, but in effect I didn't have any, since they considered the cancer a preexisting condition and wouldn't pay for anything relating to it for a year. (They wouldn't pay for Lyme disease, either, because I had had it before the policy took effect. They would only pay for conditions I didn't have.) Fortunately, I did not feel a need for serious diagnostics at that time. I had already decided that I would not use CT scans, due to radiation and toxicity from injected contrast media.

2 May 03...Energy better this AM after writing in journal last night...Did GIM with Joy today; used percussion over the belly to focus vibration; worked well. Felt energy moving, first in a circle, then in counterclockwise spiral, then in clockwise spiral at 2nd chakra.

Emotions very raw today. Tears from deep within, beginning at the uterus and coming up; chest pain during GIM; heart pain...Karen did a (yoga) set aimed at unifying mind/body/spirit and deep healing. Again, tears from deep within, about having used so much energy for others and keeping none for myself. Tonia held my hand. I felt the strength of my community around me again....

13 May 03:...Slept poorly last night; body itching & jumping and wouldn't settle down--head either. Thought I needed magnets [I had sold magnets in the early days of the practice as an aid to circulation], *but that didn't work; guess I needed Mozart.*

Feeling washed up at 54; struggling to get through a day's work. It's strange. I don't feel old or obsolete; it's merely that sometimes the body says she can't do what she's asked. Of course, in school I didn't have to do anything except the academic thing at times like these, when garbage, known and unknown, is boiling up. I can have a breakdown if I feel like it, so long as I get to bed on time and can act normal by 10 AM.

"So cut the crap," my body said. "You can't do healing and total transformation and so on while continuing to do the same old things and keeping the lid on it." The body wants to let the dragon breath out to singe everything in its path.

Many voices are giving me their opinion as to how this is going. At times it feels like a downhill slide into dissolution; is that all there is? And would getting carved up like a Christmas turkey save my life or merely alter it in many unwanted ways?

I don't think I was given the problem merely to cut out the voice of the body, but instead to let her speak.

How am I to get from here to there? I would like a closer explanation of the step known as "a miracle occurs." Probably won't get that explanation yet. (from my journal)

Cooling the hot blood of anger

In May I decided I needed to resolve that problematic old Workers' Comp case one way or the other, and filed for arbitration, while I wasn't busy dying. I had a terrible time plowing through the paperwork and figuring out what had been paid and what hadn't. And looking at it made me absolutely furious!

The "hot blood of anger" was more than a metaphor. I was running a great deal of heat, which is recorded in the bright reds and yellows and flames in the mandalas I drew during the Guided Imagery sessions at this time. The earliest ones show a smoldering, the middle ones show the flame, and the later ones show more blues and water—a cooling down. Interspersed with the high drama described in my journals are comments about writing insurance reports and so on—the sublime intermingled with the ridiculous.

Kundalini yoga has a remedy that I found helpful for the heat and probably could have used more. Sitali Pranayam, or "cooling breath," consists of breathing through a curled tongue. Karen, our yoga teacher, explains that it is "a liver and blood cleanser, reduces fever, and oxygenates the system with long, slow breathing. Calming, so good for anger. Good for hot flashes or in summer. It strengthens the parasympathetic nervous system." Two simple ways of stimulating the parasympathetics are taking a deep breath and drinking a glass of water. Sitali Pranayam is a much more focused way of achieving this same result.

On a more metaphysical level, Karen says, it "connects you with the element ether, which is how things are manifested out of the blue, and opens the throat chakra so that what you say is true." During this period, we did Sitali Pranayam frequently in yoga class. Karen has always been good at planning the yoga class according to what is needed, sometimes consciously, and sometimes simply by being open to her guidance.

Seventeen

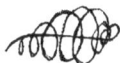

AMAS Blood Test Borderline.
Anemia Persisting. Some Improvement

June 2003

I n June, six months after the initial diagnosis, I decided to use the AMAS blood test (Antimalignin Antibody in Serum) as a means of monitoring the cancer. It was inexpensive enough ($135 at that time) for me to be able to afford, despite the fact that the insurance wouldn't pay for it. The AMAS tests the body's immune response to malignin, a protein present in the blood of anyone who has cancer. According to Oncolab, the laboratory that performs the test, an elevated antibody titer (the amount of antibody in a sample) indicates an active cancer and a good immune response, while a normal titer shows either a successfully treated cancer or a terminal one, in which case the body is too exhausted to mount a defense. I figure it is unlikely that one would be terminal and not know it.

The antibody titer came out borderline. This result echoed the state of groundlessness I found myself in. Groundlessness is rather akin to being lost in a fog. Was the borderline titer going up or down? Was I mounting a defense against cancer or wasn't I? Oncolab recommended a repeat of the AMAS, which I didn't do for financial reasons. I questioned, was this test really of any use? Dr. Abby said she didn't know of any blood test that was any better. The obvious thing to do was to get out of town again and go to Virginia Beach for another lymph cleanse and visit to the psychic. So I arranged for Heather to cover my chiropractic office two days a week and for her to pack those days full, the way I used to.

Joy and I headed for Virginia Beach, in the high season this time, and enjoyed what had come to be my ritual lunches and carrot juice at the Heritage Store. Belinda the psychic said my body was strong and said she saw me writing two books in the future, one in about two years from then and one in about seven years, and that she saw me teaching in a non-traditional manner, to small groups of about seven or so. I asked about Doc. She said, "He's a master, not just another dead person hanging around."

Shamanic Journey #2: Chicagoland

Joy had originally planned to go with me to Chicago at the end of June but decided not to, and I suspect the universe meant it so, because the trip might have taken an entirely different shape. Dr. Fran, my friend from chiropractic school, met me at O'Hare, and we stopped for dinner at a Thai restaurant to wait out the traffic. We had fortune cookies. Mine said, "You are almost there." I believe in fortune cookies. There are times when they are definitely communications from a higher source, and I thought (and still do) that this was one of those times.

Our dance card was to be quite full for that week I was in Chicagoland, where I had gone to school. The following morning, we would meet with her friends Betty and Melba for a Reiki share. That is, each one of us would take a turn on the Reiki table, receiving the hands-on healing energy—spirit-guided life force— from several Reiki practitioners at once. Melba had been dealing with breast cancer, which had metastasized to bone, and had achieved some remission with extensive use of prayer and Reiki.

The share began with the practitioners treating me. I remember their warm, supporting energy. Fran said that she "saw" a Native American spiritual guide around me and seemed somewhat puzzled at that, since she knew I hadn't felt any particular connection with Native Amencan culture at that time. During that session I had a past life recall of having hemorrhaged to death in childbirth.

"Mary [a friend who then lived in Chicago] left a message for you," Fran told me the next day. "Also, Mary Beth offered to do a hypnotherapy session with you in the early afternoon." When I called her back, Mary told me she had been working with an Apache healer, Billie Topa Tate, and suggested we call for an appointment. Both our schedule and the healer's turned out to be full, but Mary said there would be a meditation session that evening, which was open to the public; she gave us directions, and said she'd meet us there that night. The meditation was in Evanston. Mary Beth was in Oak Lawn. In between these two events, held at opposite ends of Chicagoland, we were scheduled to meet up with Virginia, an Al-Anon friend of mine, in LaGrange. So this turned out to be a day of profound healing, interspersed with frantic dashes from one end of Chicagoland to the other, as we tried to coordinate with various people over the cell phone.

Testing for the origins of the cancer

We began our sessions with Mary Beth, a hypnotherapist with whom Fran and I had done an Inner Child experiential workshop in 1990. That workshop had led to some valuable insights, and was my first inkling of how many memories can be buried in the body. Mary Beth said it was quite a tall order to try to get to the root of my problem in two hours—and it certainly was, because I found I spent almost an hour explaining just what had been happening before I got the cancer. As I listened to myself, I realized for the first time how much I had been through in the last four years or so—buying the house, Doc's illness and dying, the frantic pace of the practice from 1999 until I came down with Lyme in 2002, the battles with Workers' Comp and, mostly, coping with my mother's worsening condition, also from 1999 on, with her series of hospitalization crises starting in 2000.

It had been inevitable that I would get sick, somehow.

After a little discussion of Overeaters Anonymous (I don't remember why) and the work of Louise Hay, and a book she recommended, Mary Beth questioned my body by muscle testing my arm.

"Are you testing a theory?" she asked. The arm remained strong when she pushed down on it. "That was a definite yes."

Then she asked about when the cancer began. "Age 43?" The arm remained strong. "Age 44?" The arm remained strong. Age 44 was my last year in chiropractic school. "Age 45?"

The arm went down. I explained that that was the year I returned to New York.

"Is it to do with your father?" The arm remained strong.

"Your mother?" The arm went down.

"Go back to the time the cancer began."

So I did. In an image I saw myself just a few days short of my tenth birthday. We were having Christmas dinner. My grandmother on my father's side was with us for the holiday. I hadn't made my bed, and I don't know how or why the subject came up, but my mother exploded and in effect kicked me out of the family for the duration of dinner. Everyone else went along with her, except my grandmother, the only one who would speak to me. My grandmother's birthday was on Christmas Day, so, like me, she was a Capricorn and the mother of the astrologer aunt who later introduced me to Edgar Cayce. Of all the family members, she, my father (a Taurus) and I were the only ones who were born in earth signs. "We goats understand each other," she said. (When she died two years later, I lost one of my major supports in a family system that I perceived as a young child to be largely unfriendly, as so many children do. There seemed to be an "us-against-them" dynamic at times, consisting of me and my father versus everybody else.) I remembered talking about this Christmas incident in therapy about ten years before. I still find it hard to talk about.

Cancer created in three stages

Mary Beth suggested using neurolinguistic programming to change the impact of the experience. " Choose an image that strikes you as ludicrous and change your mother into that," she suggested. I didn't find this nearly as helpful as the simple act of bringing the incident to light.

The implications of the Christmas incident connection, to my mind, are tremendous. ("Uterus is the mother," Belinda the psychic had said in January.) The initiating event for a cancer doesn't even have to be a physical insult. A word can be enough.

Children are especially vulnerable, as rapidly growing tissues are more susceptible to cancer that can develop many years later. At the age I was then, the uterus had begun to grow.

So that was the initiating event.

It is generally thought that the development of cancer occurs in three stages: initiation, promotion, and progression. One usually has little or no control over the initiating event, but even after this has occurred, a cancer will not develop if there is no promoting event. So most efforts toward cancer prevention, such as dietary interventions, focus on preventing the promoting event, the impetus that makes the cancer happen.

It occurred to me that the constellation of events leading up to the cancer bore a great deal of similarity to a prior series of crises that had ultimately led to my undergoing five years of therapy while in chiropractic school. The chief difference was simply that the stress expressed itself physically, in the case of the cancer, rather than solely emotionally. So, in a sense, when I was diagnosed with cancer, I had a pretty good idea about how I got there; there was an air of familiarity about it. And I knew that I had survived the prior situation and come out the better for it.

My collection of crises

The collection of crises I had endured in the fall of 1988, just prior to my leaving New York for chiropractic school, included these: My mother had a heart attack; my father, who was staying with Mimi in Ohio while my mother was in the hospital for a hip replacement, developed a pulmonary embolism, and my alcoholic partner hit bottom and went into rehab. *All in about a week.* My younger sister Fran was pregnant with her son Mikie, who was born while our mother was in the nursing home. My sisters

Mimi and Janet, and I, who lived closer to my mother, developed a division of labor to cope with all this, which stood us in very good stead throughout the rest of my mother's life, and brought all four of us much closer.

It wasn't a surprise that during this time I began having panic attacks, which I have never had before or since. I spent the five years in chiropractic school putting myself back together.

My feeling is that, had I remained in Chicago and not returned to the area where my mother lived, I would not have gotten cancer, and my path would have been entirely different. As it was, my body told me that the promotion stage of the cancer occurred at age 45—when I returned to New York.

Mary Beth and I had done the almost impossible: We came up with the answer in two hours.

"I can't believe you have cancer," Mary Beth said. "You don't look it at all."

This comment of Mary Beth's illustrates the mythic perception of cancer in Western culture. Baldness, which has become a symbol of cancer, has nothing to do with cancer itself and everything to do with the conventional medical treatment of it. Extreme weight loss is either a symptom of a cancer that is very far advanced or a result of chemo- or radiation-induced nausea. It's another symptom I never had. In fact, it may be possible to have cancer brewing for many years, or remaining at a standstill, without it showing outwardly at all, depending on type and location.

Here I was, then, in Chicagoland, among old friends eager to share their healing strategies and their love and support with me. The timing worked out that we would end up doing a great deal of this work in the space of an afternoon.

A healing in a serene space

Now it was on to a whirlwind lunch stop to meet my Al-Anon friend Virginia in LaGrange, and then to Evanston to meet with Mary for the meditation at the Mystical Sciences Institute with the Apache healer Billie Topa Tate. The building was rather unusual. I think it had been originally an industrial building, which had been beautifully converted into apartments around a central courtyard, giving it a sense of light and space. I remember the flowers in particular. Billie Topa Tate's space included two floors. Upstairs were a little shop and a balcony; a stairway led downstairs to a large room around an atrium, surrounded by a kitchen and (I think) other smaller rooms. The light and space created a deep sense of calm. Mary explained to us that Billie's method of healing was a blend of the Apache and Buddhist traditions as well as other influences. Forty or fifty people made a circle around the atrium. We closed our eyes. The circle began with drumming, which vibrated through my entire body and seemed to center in the uterus in particular. Billie Topa Tate told us it was her mother's seventieth birthday, so we went around the circle, wishing happy birthday to Mama Little Wolf, who thanked us and gave us all a copy of a prayer she had written for the occasion. (This is hanging on the office wall behind me as I write.)

Billie Topa Tate then asked us to close our eyes and led us in a "Loving Kindness Meditation." We were told to focus on someone we loved. After the events taking place earlier in the day, my mother was at the top of my mind; I followed along with the meditation and was able to forgive her on the etheric level. How much harder it was to let go on the material plane, I was yet to find out.

Eighteen

Crop Walk: Are We There Yet?

Summer/Fall 2003

S o there it was. I had an answer. Now that I'd gotten the point, couldn't we dispense with the cancer now?

Not quite.

I returned home and promptly developed a dental infection—I had had twinges from it from time to time, but this time I couldn't make it go away. It was July 4 weekend, of course (the anniversary of the tick bite that gave me Lyme), so I would have to make an emergency dental appointment. I had some qualms about using my regular dentist, because he did not take the question of amalgam toxicity seriously. I had a mouth full of it, and I decided not to have any more. So I changed dentists. It turned out that the tooth in question was beyond any chance of filling with amalgam or anything else, so I debated whether to have a root canal or simply have it pulled. I had the root canal, it failed, and the tooth had to be pulled anyway. But I had an incredible surge of energy after it was gone and realized it had probably been leaking infection and toxicity into my system for some time. The dentist commented that my liver must be working pretty well, because the Novocain wore off so fast. That is because I was still doing castor oil packs daily. I had three more bad amalgam fillings removed and replaced and felt the difference immediately.

Heather was working the practice; I certainly didn't have the energy to do it. I was therefore available to do house calls for a new patient with an acute low-back problem and was comforted to see that I could still do it. Other than that, and the dental work, I spent much of July walking, sitting out in the sun, resting, and other healthy things that I had been out of the habit of doing. Joy and I decided to go to Nova Scotia and possibly Newfoundland in August, before the school year started again in September. But I had been working hardly at all and paying Heather, and money was short, so we didn't go to Newfoundland. We stopped off in Otis, Maine on the way to Nova Scotia to visit Doc's friend Kathleen in her camp by the lake on the way up and the way back. I am eternally grateful that we had the chance to spend that time with her. It turned out to be the last time I visited her there.

(Once I asked Kathleen why Doc, with all his knowledge, had not done better with his own cancer. "He didn't take his own advice," she said.)

O Canada!

We were planning to stay in the Poplar Hill schoolhouse when we got to Nova Scotia. In 1970 my mother had bought it from the neighbor diagonally across the street, a few years after the consolidation of the school district and the closing of the one-room schoolhouses in Pictou County, where it is located. I had gone there almost every summer since then. Kit, who lived across the street, had been a childhood friend of my mother's who moved to Nova Scotia in 1969 and lived there until her death in 1999. I had formed a close relationship with Kit, who was like a second mother to me, and enjoyed friendships with Barb and Vince, who helped Kit in her later years. Many of my friends in Nova Scotia were of Kit's generation and had passed on by this time, and I had lost track of several others.

The schoolhouse was a wreck when we got to Nova Scotia; it had been broken into again, more of the furniture had been stolen, and the pump didn't work. We spent a lot of time working around the place and trying to get things done, rather than enjoying the time there, which might have been a better thing to do. But I found myself overwhelmed with grief over the many losses I had sustained there, particularly Kit's death. The bleeding increased, to reflect this emotional state.

When we returned home in September, I knew I had to go back to work and didn't feel ready to. The tenant had moved out of the cottage unexpectedly at the end of June, and so I had lost that source of income, and the school tax was due at the end of the month. (I have noticed that time, tide, and taxes wait for no man or woman, and they don't wait for cancer either.) It was in no condition to rent, so I figured I would have to fix it up. Joy, an experienced carpenter, offered to help, and I gratefully accepted. We worked together on the cottage one or two evenings a week after I was done with patients for the day, though I didn't feel my energy was quite up to it.

Was I going to die? Nah.

The last Sunday in September, the day of the Crop Walk, dawned overcast, but cleared as the day wore on. Crop Walk is a nation-wide walk to raise money against world hunger, sponsored locally by Teresa's church and other churches. Teresa was involved in organizing it, and therefore participating in Crop Walk had become a tradition for The Crew. That year, Teresa was working at one of the refreshment stations, and Jean and I decided to do the walk.

In 2001, Jean had walked five miles on the River Road, a gravel road, on crutches. She was pretty sure she couldn't walk the whole thing this year and had decided to take the wheelchair, but she didn't think the wheelchair would make it on the gravel. So she decided to do the ten-mile walk over Music Mountain, because that road was paved.

I wasn't going to let her do it alone, so I did the same and caught up with her about half way through. She had sprained her wrist a few days before. She found she had to walk more than she had originally intended to, and wore out the toes of her shoes. We were the last ones in, but we finished. I found I was no more tired than I would normally expect to be after a ten-mile walk.

So was I going to die? *Nah.*

The fall went on; the cottage project turned out to be much more involved than I thought, and working at my practice and attempting to renovate it at the same time was really proving to be too much.

Work with Jean was becoming increasingly difficult, as she was realizing she needed to sell her house and move away—she had no idea where, just somewhere. Trying to accomplish anything with her in that state of depression was rather akin to swimming through glue. Jean had gone off Buprenex in July 2002, while I was in the throes of Lyme disease. She had decided this was imperative, because we were finding it almost impossible to get anyone to prescribe it any more. She had lost three pain management doctors since starting on Buprenex in 1992, and wasn't willing to shop for another one. We had also become concerned about the possible long-term health consequences of her being on a central nervous system depressant for ten years; Buprenex had not been designed for this type of use. Her orthopedist and I had both thought it would be necessary for her to go through a detox program, but she took matters into her own hands and proved us wrong, taking a weekend to drive up to Cape Cod with Teresa, returning drug-free.

Good drug, bad drug

There was both an upside and a downside to coming off the Buprenex. The good thing about a drug is that it makes it possible to tolerate the intolerable, and the bad thing about a drug is that it makes it possible to tolerate the intolerable. Since discontinuing the drug, Jean had been in more pain and had lost mobility. She had also become aware that her life as it was had become intolerable and she would have to change it. Without discontinuing the drug, and without this realization, she would have missed the chance at happiness that was to come later. But this would not have been the only consequence.

When Jean started the Buprenex in 1992, it may have saved her life by taking the edge off the pain. This was also a two-edged sword, because it permitted her to do things physically through sheer force of will that her body was not strong enough to do, and therefore may have exacerbated her injuries. It also blunted the edge of her awareness another little bit, though in comparison to other drugs I have encountered, it allowed her to function very well. A doctor I corresponded with called it "the best drug I have seen in forty years." By the summer of 2002, however, her emotional healing had progressed to the point that she needed that bit of awareness that the Buprenex had taken away. Had she not taken herself off the drug, she would not have known that she needed to move out of her house, with the many years of toxic memories it held. "If I hadn't moved out of that house," she now says, "I'd be dead." So, in 2002, remaining on Buprenex could have killed her.

One day, we were working on the right knee. I had not been receiving as many messages from the knees since I had come down with Lyme, possibly because my energy was low and partially due to Jean's depression since coming off the Buprenex.

On this occasion the right knee spoke out loudly and clearly: "Stop calling me Baby. I'm eight years old, practically grown up."

"I know where she got that," Jean said when I repeated the message. "I was nine when I started taking care of my mother."

Subtle clues from my body

I had been reading Susun Weed's *The Menopausal Years,* having decided to treat the cancer as a hormonal imbalance, which it was. The year before, chaste tree berries had been suggested to me as part of a protocol for a patient, to stop flooding, and I had taken some tablets for a while. I had become interested in them recently; this I find often happens when I need an herb or supplement at that moment. My body will clue me in in this way. This time I decided to order the berries themselves from Jean's

Greens. Susun Weed had mentioned that they were slow to act, and it would take about six months to see any change.

In my case, not exactly.

I put them in my scrambled eggs in the morning. In consistency they were like little peppercorns and very hard. Later on I broke a tooth on one. They didn't stop the flooding; they started it. Within twenty-four hours I was flooding once a day, usually in the afternoon or the early evening, complete with the emotional upheaval that usually went along with it. In short, I was a disaster.

About a week before Thanksgiving, I got a message from the universe telling me to trust, and put Teresa in the cottage, since Teresa would be losing her home and was going to need a place to live.

Nineteen

De Mortuis Nihil Nisi Bonum.
Speak Nothing but Good of the Dead

Thanksgiving 2003

For Thanksgiving, all the family were in New Canaan except for Mimi, who had just been there a few weeks before. My mother, according to Olive, her caretaker, had been asking if everybody was going to be there. She had never gained her energy back after the radiation, partly due to the radiation itself and partly due to the seizure medication they had her on. She stayed in bed during the meal, which was highly uncharacteristic, as she always wanted to be in the middle of the action and not miss a thing. Everyone took turns going into the den, where the hospital bed was, and staying with her.

Fran told me that mother had been breathing very laboriously the night before and wanted to call hospice to get them to do something. I said that was pointless. Olive said before we went to bed that she thought mother might slip away during the night. I held mother's hand before going to sleep on the floor in the adjoining room.

I woke up at about one a.m. to go to the bathroom and couldn't hear her breathing. I did a couple of chest compressions and she breathed one last time.

That was it.

I awakened Olive, who called the funeral home and the hospice nurse. At about 3 a.m. the people from the funeral home came and shepherded us into the other room while they took her away.

No matter how prolonged, or how expected, it seems to me that there is always an abrupt quality, an element of surprise when someone dies, "the surprise of the inevitable," as Joanne Greenberg says in *I Never Promised You A Rose Garden.* I felt unprepared for it.

We decided to have a brief service within a few days and then do a memorial in the spring. Fran and I went over to the funeral home to choose the casket (I knew my mother didn't like blond wood). To put in the casket with her, Fran chose three small items—a ceramic cardinal she had painted while at Sharon Health Care, a pack of cigarettes, and her little portable ashtray. This seemed appropriate and had its element of humor. There seems to be a lot of arranging and a lot of deciding that goes into funerals. Fran and Olive were invaluable at this time.

Mimi, who was in charge of accounting, gave $10,000 to each of us. I was yet to see quite how neatly the universe had arranged everything.

Twenty

Broken Leg. Time Out

January 2004

"The best-laid plans of mice and men gang aft aglae.' –Robert Burns

I don't remember December very well. Months later I found an Independent Medical Examiner report dated December 5 denying further care to one of my Comp patients. In fact, there is nothing independent about an Independent Medical Examiner. He or she is hired by the insurance carrier to state that the patient no longer needs care and to justify this in any way, possible or improbable. Apparently the insurance carrier also forgot about it for a few months, as well, because I kept on getting paid.

Hummy and Jean worked on the cottage bathroom, now that there was the inheritance to pay for it, before Hummy went south for the winter. The financial pressure was off, at least for the moment. Jean was involved in the last throes of housecleaning before turning over her house to the buyer and also heading south—she didn't know where, just that she had to go someplace far away and warm. Early in January Teresa rented a truck and Hummy and I moved her into my cottage, while Jean stayed at her house to finish the housecleaning. I told Teresa that she could stay in the cottage through the winter. She had several applications in for housing, all in Connecticut, but we had no idea when any of them would come through.

The one-year waiting period on what I would come to call "the stupid insurance" covering me would expire on January 1. The family would also stop paying for it at that time. So I scheduled the first ultrasound for January 31. Weather that January consisted of alternating thaws and freezes; snow would fall, melt a little, and freeze again. Late in the month, Jean headed for wherever she was going, which turned out to be Concord, North Carolina. On January 31, I went to the bank before going to Sharon Hospital for the ultrasound, and slipped on the ice. Not being inclined to sit in the snow, I got up and started limping home. I got as far as the office across the street, where I sat down and worked on the leg. Once I had sat down, I found I could no longer bear weight on it at all.

Oops.

Jean answers the call of spirit

I phoned Teresa, who was at the cottage now, and she took me over to the hospital, where I was supposed to have been going anyway. After taking a number of pictures, they decided that I had broken the fibula (the smaller bone on the outside of the lower leg) in two places, one a bit below the knee and one at the ankle.

I suppose anything worth doing is worth doing thoroughly. They decided the ultrasound could wait.

Jean showed up at the emergency room, having just arrived from North Carolina in the wee small hours of the morning. She had been having trouble with her neck and back and had been planning to come back north the following week to see me— "But,' she said, "I was told, 'GO NOW,' and I said, 'All right, Lord.'" She had driven up north, hoping I would be able to adjust her the next day. I have never been so glad to see anyone. I ended up with a cast up to the knee—the orthopedist figured that would slow me down quite enough, and not having the knee cast would keep it from stiffening. They prescribed 800 mg. of ibuprofen; Jean figured rightly that this was far too much, since I hadn't taken any prescription or over-the counter pain medication since 1991 or prior, and so she picked up some 200 mg. tablets at the drugstore.

Jean tells me that she and Teresa dragged me up the stairs into the house on a coat (I have some vague recollection of this). They settled me on the couch in the front room, Barbara's office, for the time being. Olive was still living at my mother's condo in New Canaan. The orthopedist had told me I would be in a cast for eight weeks, so we called Olive to ask if she wanted to be employed again. She said she would be available on Sunday (it was Friday). Jean stayed until Toni and Olive arrived with a twin bed to be set up in the reception room, and then headed south again.

31 January:...I am a beached whale. What does a beached whale do? Can't swim, can't clean house, can't treat patients.

I am relatively well stocked for invalidism, using Jean's wheelchair, my mother's commode, a walker. The shower chair will come in handy when I am wheeled into the bathroom to attempt to wash...What does a beached whale do? The body is useless, so the life of a beached whale has to take place in the mind. (from my journal)

Laid up and frustrated

I was appalled at how little I could do. The crutches I had used in 1988 for torn ligaments in my right ankle were too tall for me now, and I didn't have the upper body strength to manage them anyway, with a lump of lead hanging on my right leg. This was a graphic indication of how much conditioning I had lost since I moved out of New York. So I had to do all my navigation with the walker and the wheelchair. I took 400 mg. of ibuprofen for three nights and never touched it again.

A couple of days later, Kathleen stopped in and offered to pick me up lunch at KJ's. It was the last time I saw her alive.

Olive and I settled into a comfortable routine. I was ensconced in the reception room, the only place downstairs where the bed would fit. Therefore I had to be presentable by the time the patients came in. We arranged for Heather to work for me twice a week, and Barbara was still seeing her own clients three days a week. Teresa came in three days a week for errands and office work. So not only was I unable to loaf, I was reminded of exactly how much non-income-producing work has to be done to maintain the practice. After supper, Olive and I would watch a movie together before bedtime. Probably neither of us had watched this many movies in the previous ten years.

Jean returned north in ten days' time, just in time for my first doctor's office visit and my first attempt at getting out of the house. This trip was not to the orthopedist, which would have made sense, but to the local clinic that served as my "primary care physician" under the rules of the stupid insurance. They told me I had to see them first to get a referral to the orthopedist, because the insurance company said so. It was quite clear to me what the problem was, and I was quite sure I wasn't in cardiac arrest or anything, but they had to make me go in there to take my blood pressure (which Olive or I could easily have done at home). The fact that it was still February and icy at times made me exceedingly nervous, and the huge expenditure of effort this required, to no purpose, annoyed me greatly.

After managed care wasted my time and the stupid insurance company's money on this foolishness, I subsequently received a $300 bill for this visit, three separate line items at $100 apiece. The insurance had paid $27 on each of them. I was charged a $20 co-pay.

A description of dying well

Getting in and out of the house that first time was a major production; we called in a strong male friend to help out. Getting down the stairs, while no picnic, was not so bad; getting up required my sitting down on one of the steps, having someone run around and put a low beach chair at the top so that I could sit in that and get my legs up to the second step. Then someone would run and fetch the wheelchair; I would stand up on the second step and sit in the wheelchair, then I was ready to go. All of this became progressively easier as I got stronger. Olive (or Teresa) and I got pretty good at it.

Our next trip out was to Kathleen's funeral. Her family told me it had been a quick and easy death—the MRI had come out badly on Tuesday, Wednesday she was in pain, and Thursday she was gone.

My journal for that period reads:

...She did not cling to life beyond possibility, neither did she hasten to end it before its time. This is dying well.

This doesn't stop my tears at being left behind.

I got stronger, and getting around got easier. We ran through Teresa's movies and started on Dorothy's. In the evening Olive and I would sit around the supper table and she would tell me about her mother's knowledge and use of herbs in Jamaica. Olive became famous at the thrift shop in Sharon for the outfits she could put together for two dollars. She was always well turned out when she went to church! I like to think that helping me was a vacation of sorts for her, too, because she knew she could go out and leave me alone, and she didn't have to worry about my having a medical emergency while she was out. She also didn't have to make sure I ate—I can usually do that—and she didn't have to monitor my pills. I took care of the supplements myself, and there were no medications. I ate well and healthily and didn't gain any weight. When I woke up to use the commode at night I would do my Tai Chi on it before going back to bed. On Tuesday mornings she took me over to the healing service. Nigel commented that I was getting "holy rest," and I had to concede that he was right.

Two months passed in this rather pleasant way. By the end of the first month, Teresa and I were going upstairs (I on my butt, she on her feet) to do the bookkeeping on the computer. We used the beach chair trick at the top of the stairs. The cast came off in late March. I had originally thought I might try to rehab the leg myself, but soon realized I had grossly overestimated my energy level. Because the fall had occurred on the bank's property, the bank's insurance paid for Olive and for Heather's and Teresa's expenses, and ultimately for physical therapy, as well.

Shortly after the cast came off, Olive went back to New Canaan. The universe had made sure she was available at the right time. I could not have recovered nearly so well without her. Jean,

Teresa and Heather had also been there exactly when I needed them—and the funds were available to pay them.

Once more, the universe knew better than I did what had to happen and arranged the choreography flawlessly.

Twenty-one

"Consistent with invasive carcinoma; ovaries normal; no ascites." AMAS normal. No anemia.

April 2004

In April, my sisters Mimi and Fran planned a memorial gathering for my mother in New Canaan. It did not take place at a church, but instead at the Historical Society. A friend of Fran's catered a tea, and many friends attended and spoke. It was beautifully done, which I can say without being egotistical, since I can take absolutely no credit for it.

I had the ultrasound done in April and promptly rewarded myself with another Virginia Beach trip with Tonia. In my opinion, this was by far the most pleasant way to await results— by not thinking about it at all. I was not getting around well yet, and still had to use the walker occasionally. So we headed down and let the universe do the guiding. Tonia turned off the highway in Lewes at a place that advertised chelation therapy; she wanted to check it out. They also stocked the herbs for the Hulda Clark parasite cleanse, and we each bought some, since I had been thinking about doing it, anyway.

We stayed at the Schooner, had our ritual Lymph Cleanse at the A.R.E., had fun book shopping and drinking our carrot juice at the Heritage Store, and tried to make an appointment with Belinda the psychic, who was unavailable. We scheduled with Maria instead. Having been to Nova Scotia with Joy the previous summer and seen the poor condition of the schoolhouse, I had this issue at the forefront of my mind: What should I, or we, do about the schoolhouse?

Maria said she saw the work being done with someone else's money—"maybe a grant of some kind. I think it could be fun." I asked about my health. She said, "The body is strong."

Upon our return from Virginia Beach, Teresa shared great news. She had been accepted at the Station Place apartment complex in Canaan, Connecticut. This was perfect for her, because it was in the middle of town. Canaan was close enough to all of us so that she wouldn't feel she was moving away from us, yet also far enough away that she felt she was making a fresh start. Our original deal was for her to stay in the cottage through the winter; however, I had had no intention of asking her to leave when spring came if she did not have a place to go. I didn't have to think about it. The universe provided. By the time she left, I could get up and down stairs, do the errands and work the practice on my own.

Another salute to the body's intelligence

I did do about a month's worth of physical therapy after getting back from Virginia Beach. In comparison to the previous June, the bloodwork was outstanding. Olive had done her caretaking job well. I was rested, although not necessarily by my own choice. Hemoglobin was up to 13.9 from 11.1. RDW, at 16.0, showed that the body was making a large effort to recoup the blood loss. RDW is a measure of the variation in blood cell sizes. It can mean a large number of immature (or "band") red blood cells, which are larger than mature ones. It can also mean a combination of iron-deficiency anemia (cell size too small) and B 12 anemia (cell size too large because red blood cells cannot reproduce properly).

This ultrasound gave us vital information. Dr. Abby explained that endometrial cancer metastasizes to the ovaries first, and the normal ovaries indicated that it hadn't metastasized. She also asked me if I'd had a prior ultrasound for comparison. "No," I said, and she appeared puzzled, as the uterus was a normal size. What usually happens in an "untreated" endometrial cancer is that the uterus will keep getting bigger and bigger and sometimes may even burst. I had been flooding on and off for two years at this point, so I had a fair idea where the excess had gone. Flooding, which had been less during the Lyme disease, also lessened during the healing process with my leg, for which I was duly grateful. I took my hat off once more to the intelligence of the body.

I started the parasite cleanse the same day I saw Dr. Abby, and continued for the full three weeks. It consisted of wormwood, black walnut hulls, and cloves; it gave me gas, as I expected, but I felt an upsurge of energy afterward. I also got a helpful laundry hint from Dr. Hulda Clark's book: using peroxide to clean bloodstains. It saves a lot of scrubbing.

Taking care of old business

In June, I finally got called to Kangaroo Court on that unresolved Comp case, the one I had decided needed to be resolved one way or the other. It was only a little more than a year since I had put in for a hearing (I had taken a little time off from dying to do that). I was still walking with a stick; getting around was an effort, let alone preparing a case. I hadn't the slightest idea what they were after. There was such a morass of material, and it made me so furious every time I looked at it, that it was almost impossible for me to focus on it. I had last seen that patient in November 2000, less than two months after we had allegedly "won" the case. Two years of wrangling in court had ended up gaining me the right to treat her twice a month, when what she really needed was twice a week. Two months after that, she had ended up in the hospital with gall bladder surgery—or was it appendix that time? No, it was gall bladder, because I thought at the time the problem was almost certainly iatrogenic, caused by medical treatment.

So I was called into a gray, windowless room in a gray, windowless building, with two gray old men sitting on a dais. The insurance carrier had a staffer or two going through stacks of paper—I guess they pay people to do precisely this—while I had to take half a day from my practice to attend this Kangaroo Court, having paid forty dollars for the privilege of attempting to collect for work I had done four years before. The two gray men clearly had not read the volumes of material I had laboriously put in the record, only the report of the carrier's hired gun. Leafing through the material I had in the file later, I found a very well-written reexam report I had written as a rebuttal two weeks after the IME report. This should have been available to the two gray old men conducting the hearing, as I had sent it to the Comp board at that time. I spoke and was interrupted, and never did get a chance to present the material I had brought. I did remark that I had had Lyme disease, cancer and a broken leg since I last saw the patient, but I forgot to mention that my mother had also died.

Tell me again, who was paying for this hearing, or rather non-hearing?

On returning home, I was grateful for the lush green of the trees, for the privilege of living and working in a beautiful place, not in a gray dead building with gray old men. And I decided never to submit to such an indignity again.

Learning more about bloodwork

June must have been a busy month. I remember sitting at KJ's, going through the mail one day when I saw another flyer for a Standard Process seminar on lipids (fats). Not thinking lipids a very sexy topic, I had let it go the first time, but the universe told me to take another look. (Actually, lipids *are* a sexy topic; all of the sex hormones are derived from cholesterol, as well as the adrenal hormones.) The seminar was to be given by Lynne August, MD, who had developed a computerized blood test evaluation to get better information out of standard bloodwork, to determine how to create optimal health, rather than simply treat disease. I had evaluated bloodwork in school and knew the basics of it, but I definitely felt there was a lot more that I could learn on this topic.

I put the mail aside to finish the book I was reading, *Appetites,* by Geneen Roth. At the end of the Acknowledgments section I read, "And to Lynne August, MD, for saving my life."

Thus spake the universe. I did as I was told and attended the seminar, which was a revelation. It was on lipids—catabolic and anabolic, according to the definitions of Dr. Emanuel Revici, with whom Lynne had done research. Dr. Revici had been working with anabolic (sterols) and catabolic (fatty acids) lipids. The "lipid defense" is designed to be an oscillation between these two—first the catabolic action tears down damaged tissue, then the anabolic stops the teardown and rebuilds. As long as the two are in balance, there is health; if one dominates the other, it not only does not solve the original problem, but creates others. He had devised a number of unique lab tests to study this and had been applying it to help determine the correct dosing of chemotherapy or radiation to individual patients.

The cancer establishment apparently found this too far out, or too labor-intensive, and still does not individualize treatment in this way. Like many pioneers in the field, Dr. Revici made it into the American Cancer Society's *Unproven Methods of Cancer Management*. Ralph Moss, Ph.D, comments in *The Cancer Industry,* "Merely including a scientist's name on this list has the effect of damning the researcher's work and putting the tag of quackery on him and his efforts." (p.98)

Lynne also discussed hydration and electrolytes. I saw that here there might be a tool for me to use to figure out my nutritional needs more precisely. Besides, I felt that we spoke the same language. I don't feel that way in professional circles very often.

A clear energy field

2004 was not a big year for travel, although I did make it to Newfoundland for Marlene and Bob's wedding in July. Late in August, Dr. Fran from Chicago and I went to a qigong conference in Lake Geneva, Wisconsin; early in the conference I slipped on some wet leaves and sprained my ankle again. This inhibited my mobility at the conference but, upon returning to Fran's house, I wrapped it in a comfrey leaf, which brought the swelling down and facilitated healing. She also arranged an appointment with John, her acupuncturist friend in Evanston.

"You're doing better than you think," he said, and told me he found no trace of the cancer in my energy field. John talked about an Amish healer in Indiana with whom he had been studying, and we had a conversation about treating candida. That afternoon he also had a patient in the office who had had chemo. They were talking about "chemo brain"—an experience I was perfectly willing to skip.

Flooding was an on-again, off-again thing during this period. I don't remember being particularly bothered by it. Then, in late October, all the family went to Washington, DC for a cousin's wedding. (These occasions have been great opportunities for us to get together with our cousins and get to know each other once again. We've run out of weddings for the time being, and will have to think of another excuse to keep up the tradition.)

I was up all night flooding and watching a program about World War II on television. I mention that because the emotional tone is similar. Flooding episodes bring up all kinds of buried emotional garbage—that's what they're for, after all. They provoke insomnia, self-hatred for no particular reason, a review of all sorts of large and small mistakes, and so on. It lasts as long as it lasts, usually several hours, and then it's over—much better! So watching a TV documentary about World War II bombers was as good a thing to be doing as any, during such a time.

I remember this so well because it was the last major flood I had. I've arbitrarily decided that it was my last menstrual period.

Why not? I had still been having menstrual cycles, after a fashion, for a while after the cancer diagnosis, though the cyclical nature became obscured by the vehemence of the flooding.

My sister Janet and I had a quiet, easygoing Thanksgiving for the first anniversary of my mother's death. That was fine with me.

Twenty-two

"Decreasing size of the uterus." AMAS, Pap normal. No anemia. RDW down

December 2004

This ultrasound result was quite clearly not what was medically expected, though it made perfect sense to me, after the amount of flooding I had just experienced. "Did you have surgery?" the ultrasound tech asked me. No, I had not. I had simply done my best to support the body in taking care of the situation. The lower RDW (variation in red blood cell size) meant to me that the body wasn't struggling as hard to make up for the loss of blood, yet numbers were staying up reasonably well. I continued to feel that Olive's ministrations, particularly her excellent cooking, with particular regard for good nutrition, were largely responsible for the major improvement in bloodwork between June 2003 and April 2004. Despite two months of enforced inactivity, I had not gained weight. I was now maintaining on my own and working the practice.

I felt that it was time for celebration.

February 2005 was a good time for a Virginia Beach run. This was the first long trip I had made alone since March 2002.

Early in April, once the weather was better, I organized a potluck and talk at Souler Power Academy for friends, local doctors who might be interested, and members of the Business Women's Network. It turned out that I was so busy organizing the potluck and making sure everyone would have something to eat that I barely had time to do more than make a couple of sketchy notes for the talk. Dona and I scheduled it for two successive Tuesday evenings, this being the night that the Business Women's Network usually met. The night before the first talk, I had supper at the local Chinese restaurant and got the following fortune cookie:

"You will be sharing great news with the people you love."

The universe had spoken again.

Speaking out about my process

There were about thirty-five people at the first session and twelve at the second. None of the doctors showed up. I found that I had a lot more than one evening's worth of material to cover. Both were lively gatherings with a lot of well-considered questions and comments.

Tonia ran a video camera to record the second one. I was quite pleased at how it went, though the tape showed me that I needed to brush up on my public speaking skills.

By this time, walking was becoming slightly less of a chore, though my gait still wasn't quite right. That small bit of dorsiflexion (the ability to bend the foot up) I lost in the right ankle after breaking my leg had a much greater effect than I would have thought. Because of it, I also lost some extension in the sacroiliac joint, couldn't bend the knee quite normally on toe-off, and the lumbar paraspinal muscles on the right worked harder than those on the left. The right leg was still weak. I knew I needed to strengthen it.

Walking up the hill was no longer strenuous enough exercise to satisfy me, and I also felt that increasing exercise would help the liver and straighten out my hormones. I considered joining the Millbrook Training Center again, because they had a pool (I had quit in 2001, both for financial reasons and because of the bleeding). However, it turned out that it would cost more than I was willing to pay, so I joined Curves, which was right in town. I could do an entire exercise routine there in the time it would take to get to Millbrook and back.

Curves was exactly what I needed. I did the Health Equations Blood Test Evaluation for the first time in late July, just before joining Curves. Dr. Lynne August asks for a measurement of the abdomen as an inexpensive way of evaluating liver function. After a couple of months at Curves I had lost nine pounds and six inches around the abdomen.

Areas of concern on the first blood test evaluation were hydration, calcium activity, and digestive function.

In September I went to Nova Scotia again to deal with the schoolhouse. I was pleasantly surprised to see it hadn't fallen down yet, but was pretty sure it would unless I did something about it. Barb and Vince had a friend who did foundation work, so I negotiated with him to get the foundation done, which consisted of moving the house, putting a bed of gravel under it, and blocking it up with pressure-treated wood and concrete block. Arranging anything meant lots of running back and forth to the Tourist Bureau to make phone calls, which was frustrating and a waste of time. I knew something would have to be done about that and priced cell phones and land lines, ultimately deciding that the cheapest and easiest way to cope with it was to put in a land line.

Learning at a school for clairvoyants

October brought another family wedding, this time in San Francisco. Mary from Chicago had moved to Stockton and chauffeured all of us around town. We had a delightful time playing tourists. A friend of my sister Mimi's taught at a school for clairvoyants in San Francisco—where students gave twenty-minute readings for ten dollars one evening per week—and arranged for us to go there. I asked my psychic about my health. "You're fine," she said. "The way that you handle it is like tuning up a car—you run it for a while, then you tinker with it for a while." Her comment about doctors was, "You don't trust them." She came up with the car analogy with no prompting from me, and indeed, when I was younger, I spent a good deal of time tuning up the various old cars I drove, so this was quite accurate. So was the remark about doctors, for reasons I have already explained.

November was the 35th anniversary celebration of the Two Way Street Coffee House in Illinois, where I had played and listened to folk music while in chiropractic school. So of course I had to go to that—Dr. Fran and I put on our dancing shoes.

As I write this, I realize how much of the latter part of 2005 was about travel and getting in shape. Sometime in there I had become less vigilant about the carrot juice and castor oil packs. I figured that I was getting enough fresh greens in the summer from Sharon's son Bill, who was growing them and selling them at the store. Since the bleeding was so much less, I also was not paying quite as much attention to getting the heavy protein. I was having a wonderful time and feeling reasonably well, so I wasn't worrying about keeping up the protocol very much.

Twenty-three

"Contains a diffusely heterogeneous mass"

December 2005

The ultrasound report that came back this time was not what I expected. It read:

".... The uterus contains a diffusely heterogeneous mass, around which there is a very thin rim of normal-appearing myometrium. The diameter of this mass is 4 mm. Both ovaries are normal. There is no free fluid. The uterus overall measures 8.6x5.2x5.9 cm. [3.39"x 2.05"x 2.32"] The endometrial mass appears to have increased somewhat in size, when compared to the previous exam."

So what the heck was that? Dr. Abby didn't have a clue, and neither did I. This ultrasound had been read by a different radiologist than the previous two. I was puzzled by the increasing size of the mass in the middle. According to the previous radiologist, there hadn't been one at all. So I decided I could make up an answer, and that's what I did. This was my movie, after all. I decided I liked the thin rim of normal-appearing myometrium (the muscular layer of the uterus, below the endometrium) and ran with that as a positive piece of news. This indicated to me that the myometrium, at least part of which had been destroyed, was rebuilding itself. The "no free fluid," equivalent to "no ascites" in previous reports, indicates that the liver was not in trouble, as free fluid in the abdomen is a sign of liver failure. So this was a Good Thing. But ideally, there should not have been a mass in the middle at all, and the endometrium and myometrium should have been distinguishable from each other by the type of sound signal, as opposed to being "heterogeneous."

I did figure it might be time to induce some bleeding again, just in case the diffusely heterogeneous mass wasn't something it ought to be. I muscle tested the chaste tree berries again, and the body said yes. But this time they didn't appear to do a thing.

The cure: dropping stupid insurance

I didn't feel any sicker, neither did I have any sort of foreboding, but I was a little disconcerted. Jenny the acupuncturist and I decided to do the triangle again, a needle pattern on the abdomen we had used in the past to induce or increase bleeding and relieve blood stagnation. With all our efforts, it took about a month to move anything. Then there was a brief flood, and the bleeding slacked off to almost nothing. It was late February before I saw Dr. Abby again. The Pap smear came out fine, but my blood pressure was something like 210/100 and didn't come down when she repeated it. I decided on a three-point program to bring it down: add extra magnesium at night, go back to drinking a lot of Goddess Tea, and drop the stupid insurance.

Dropping the stupid insurance was the cure. I would then be able to order my own tests, as I had legally been entitled to all along, but since the stupid insurance was an HMO, if I ordered the tests, they wouldn't pay for them. To my mind, this was not only giving my power away, but paying a bunch of incompetents for the privilege. It was impossible to run the practice in the black and still pay for the stupid insurance, since, for health reasons, I no longer had the option of adding new patients if money got tight. What would I use the stupid insurance for anyway? Not for cancer treatment; I had already established that. Not for heart disease; I don't like the medical model for treating heart disease. Not for digestive disorders; I could probably take care of that as well myself. I was using it to pay for monitoring. However, if I paid for all the tests and visits out of pocket, it would still come to less than the stupid insurance.

So what was it buying me, apart from a lot of annoyance and frustration? I couldn't afford annoyance and frustration—this is what drove my blood pressure up in the first place. I decided to eat the risk of medical emergency—the truth is that there is no real protection from that. I could best stack the cards in my favor by using my money to enjoy life and promote health, not buy insurance.

Jean had flown south to North Carolina and was having severe back and knee trouble again by sometime in January. Her shoulder was getting worse, and the wear and tear on it from the many round trips wasn't helping any. She returned north and began looking for an apartment. Something affordable with a ground floor access is not easy to find in this area, and nothing she looked at seemed to work out. She was in a classic double bind—she couldn't tolerate the cold up here, and she couldn't find anyone to treat her in North Carolina. "I timed him," she said of the chiropractor she had seen in North Carolina. "It was five minutes from the time I walked into the office to the time I walked out." She was getting depressed and frustrated and, I have to admit, so was I, because we really weren't getting anywhere.

But the universe was at work again.

She finally found a place, a basement apartment that was tiny, but it wouldn't be ready until later in the spring. Her lease in North Carolina wasn't up until May, so she thought she might as well go back there.

Hummy had sold his house in the fall of 2005 and was in Greensboro, North Carolina. He called Jean up and they became a couple on Valentine's Day.

She certainly wasn't expecting it. But it was perfect for both of them. They hit the road and didn't come back north until late May.

Twenty-four

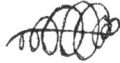

AMAS Normal. Bloodwork Improving. Why Don't I Feel Terrific?

Summer/Fall 2006

Spring was rainy. Anyone who was prone to sinus trouble had it worse than ever, and I was no exception. It wasn't absolutely terrible, but it didn't go away, either. I had gone to Virginia Beach for the Lymph Cleanse and a session with Belinda the psychic in late March. The Manual Lymphatic Drainage brought up a host of little flashing pains out of all proportion to the force used, this being an extremely gentle technique, especially as practiced by Elaine, who had studied it in Austria with Doctor Vodder. My sore right arm was considerably improved afterward, since pain seems to have a lot to do with fluid retention and lymph stagnation, which in turn causes ischemia.

I'm not quite sure what questions I had in mind to ask Belinda, and it didn't matter, because my mother showed up in spirit at the reading, so anything premeditated was out the window.

I hadn't realized that I was still harboring such a measure of guilt and discomfort around my mother's last days. Belinda said my mother was still tired and needed rest—"and kind of pissy," she added. "She wants to be sure that I respect her. I have to keep apologizing." I said that I felt badly because I had not handled the end well. Belinda said, "She says that's OK; she isn't feeling it. She says she didn't always do that well, either."

Why don't they get it?

Belinda went on to report: "She says you were always low-maintenance and handled the family situation well." We talked a bit about parents and children, about the generational differences, and what is sometimes our impatience—*Why don't they get it?* "But my daughter probably says the same thing about me," Belinda said. She then told me there were a number of "them," disembodied spirits, in the room. "They're just standing there watching. It's a little unnerving sometimes." I didn't see them, and I don't, but since I perceive things that other people don't, I have no trouble with the concept that someone else sees things I don't.

The rest of the spring must have been busy, because I don't remember it very well. I was still struggling with the numbness in my right arm, and I didn't get my taxes done on time.

Jean arrived back in mid-June, suntanned and glowing from two months on the road with Hummy. She said she loved the 105-degree heat in Arizona. Unfortunately, she had slipped on oil in a hotel parking lot and (possibly) broken her right wrist.

The bleeding was negligible by this time, and I had stopped the Lyte Cl solution, not feeling the need for it. That is an electrolyte solution Dr. Lynne August had recommended for improving my digestive function and raising the low chloride noted on the previous evaluation. Jenny was always busy, or I was always busy, and we didn't see each other for acupuncture for about two months. In late July I planned to get the AMAS and another Health Equations analysis done and then take off for Nova Scotia. I got a strong message that I needed to go—NOW! I had some patients living in abusive situations at that time, and the stuckness and hopelessness I was picking up from them was taking my energy down to a dangerously low level.

Unfortunately, the lab had forgotten to order the dry ice needed for shipping the blood sample for the AMAS, so that had to wait until after my return.

"Resting" in Nova Scotia

I was a mess when I left for Nova Scotia. My right wrist and thumb had started bothering me, and I had strained my right knee again, going down a hill by the house. This sort of thing is likely to happen at times when my energy is compromised. When I arrived at Poplar Hill, there were huge ruts in the driveway and I couldn't pull in. The telephone company, scheduled for Wednesday, didn't arrive until Thursday and couldn't finish hooking up the phone until Friday. The damage from the leaky roof didn't seem to be too bad.

The first two or three days it was just as hot as it had been in New York before I left, so the only thing to do was to go to Toney River beach and watch the snails and the jellyfish, who were abundant that week. The River John Days festival happened to be going on just after I arrived, so I paid a visit to the Lismore Sheep Farm and tried unsuccessfully to catch up with Vince and Barb at the parade.

Eventually, we did manage to connect. Vince told me he had asked someone to come in to look at the Mountain Road woodlot, as I had asked him to, and estimated there was about $10,000 worth of timber on it. "There's a stand of white spruce, mostly at the back," he said, "it's past its prime and starting to die off. If you're going to do anything with it, you'll have to do it now." There was a logger working on the McKay Road at that time, just across from where our woodlot was located. If we made the connection, he could log it almost immediately, without incurring the extra expense of bringing in his heavy equipment from somewhere else. Vince brought the logger over to talk to me, and he said he would take a look at the woodlot and give me an idea of what was on it. After looking at the lot he explained that the trees he saw there were about sixty or sixty-five years old, the natural life span of white spruce. "It's going to die anyway," he said of the stand. "You can't save it. In another two years, nobody will be willing to log it."

Mimi's name was on the title for the property, so I called her that night and explained the situation. She agreed that logging it was the obvious thing to do, and so I arranged for the logger to fax her the contract in Iowa. (Without fax machines, this transaction would never have taken place.) There was still some cleanup to be done on the foundation, so I arranged for that, too. I spent much of the trip meeting with this one and that one and arranging for this and that. Vince had a friend who was a roofer who said he would come over and look at the schoolhouse and give me an estimate. Fortunately the weather had cooled off, and I decided to take Sunday to go to the flea market, go to Melmerby Beach (this is more open water than Toney River, which is on the Northumberland Strait), then drive up along the mini-Trail to Antigonish.

Another message: Slow down

It was my goal to accomplish absolutely nothing that day, which I managed to do admirably.

I seemed to be tired a lot that trip. Probably one reason was that the ground around the schoolhouse had been plowed up with the foundation work and walking on it was difficult, exacerbating the right knee problem. Shortly before I left, I had found that my last pair of walking shoes were worn to the point of throwing my knee out. And I seemed to be back and forth to the outhouse an awful lot, despite not drinking tea any more. (The urgency was reduced, however.) I didn't even think about the bleeding when I went swimming. This was wonderful!

So the proceeds from the logging would pay for the roof. ("The work on the schoolhouse will be done with someone else's money," Maria the psychic had said.) Similarly, the foundation had been paid for by the unexpected sale of Hedgeville, another property I owned, the year before. On Thursday I overdid it, having spent the afternoon shingling and then going to the gym. So, predictably, my back went out. I interpreted this as the usual message to slow down. I did get the shingling done and a coat of primer on before it rained.

I had intended to leave Nova Scotia on Saturday, but I did not have the energy. As it turned out, the roofer came by and gave me the estimate for shingling the roof. While he was there, Bernadette visited, whom I had not seen since 1994. She said she was on the way to a potluck and a wicked croquet match in Cape John, and would I like to come along? My back was still pretty sore and I couldn't sit for long, but I said I might stop by later, which is what I did. I missed the wicked croquet match but made new connections in the community. I felt the universe was giving me a "go ahead" message about keeping the schoolhouse.

I didn't leave until quite late on Sunday. It was a holiday weekend, which I hadn't counted on. When I pulled into Sussex, New Brunswick, at 11:30 p.m. looking for a place to spend the night, I was told there was a golf tournament on and I wouldn't find anything. So I pushed on to Saint John and arrived there about 1 a.m. I could barely walk when I got out of the car, my back had stiffened up so. In the morning I struggled my way through the Tai Chi set, which helped considerably, until I sat too long at breakfast and it seized up again.

Same message, different messenger

Traffic was backed up as I pulled into St. Stephen, on the Canadian side of the border. I assume that people were returning from the holiday. I decided not to sit in traffic, and stopped at Tim Horton's for a cup of tea (my first caffeine of the whole trip) and a muffin. It had been foggy, and I was tired. When I had finished the tea and the muffin, the car wouldn't start. I had left the lights on.

The universe had spoken again. I wasn't ready to go back yet. Cars were parked on either side, so I would have to wait until one or the other car moved in order to be able to reach the battery with the jumper cables. There was no better thing to do than take care of myself while I waited, so I alternately did the Tai Chi set, sat, walked around, and felt much better, having decided to drive back toward Grand Manan and take the ferry there if it happened to time out right. I also wanted to pick up some dulse to take home, which I hadn't stopped for on the way to St. Stephen.

So did I get it yet about being fully where I was?

It seemed a long time before either of the cars moved. Finally, the owner of one of them came out and I asked if he could give me a boost. He said no, he couldn't; he'd blown his alternator the last time he'd done it, but suggested I ask the owner of the half-ton truck over there.

I did, and he did, and the car started immediately. I had to put a charge on the battery again, so I drove back toward Grand Manan, got gas, and picked up the dulse. I just missed the ferry (the clock in the car had stopped, of course, when the battery died), but that was OK. I drove around and took pictures of things and ate another delicious fish dinner and had a fine time.

And my back didn't hurt any more.

I crossed the border when I was good and ready and headed down the "Airline," Route 9. It was getting dark, and as I approached Bangor, the National Weather Service kept interrupting the interesting program I was listening to with severe thunderstorm warnings for the area I was driving into. I had thought about trying to go past Bangor to Augusta, but didn't.

Bloodwork looking good, insurance not so much

The thunderstorm never materialized, except for a few lightning flashes and a bit of rain that started as I pulled into the motel. I remember waking up in the night with my heart pounding from the two cups of Canadian tea I had had at supper.

Bloodwork results had come in on the fax machine when I returned home, so I faxed them to Dr. Lynne August at Health Equations. Offhand, they looked pretty good—electrolyte balance was better and calcium was improved. Serum iron and serum ferritin were up. When I spoke to Lynne, however, she pointed out that glucose was slightly elevated (100, as opposed to the usual 93), uric acid was up another point, digestive index was down—"and you're still iron deficient," she said. "You have more RBCs, and they're smaller, so you have more oxygen-carrying capacity. RDW is down" (which I had noticed, meaning that I wasn't working as hard to make new red blood cells, but still managing to keep the numbers up).

So why didn't I feel terrific? I still seemed to be tired a lot and had a low-grade depression, and I didn't feel as though my "vacation" was enough. Lynne suggested starting Malic Acid again and resuming the electrolytes, as well as some enzymes and a *Saccharomyces* product from Standard Process to help with the elevated uric acid, which she said was fungal in origin.

I was returning home to continue my efforts to get paid on two of my Comp cases, for one thing. It seemed that everything I attempted had to be done over before it achieved any result. I was looking at the drain on my energy this was causing and realized that I had to cut down treatment time on these cases. I had already notified the patients that I would not fight their cases before the Comp Board—that they were responsible for anything their insurer didn't pay. The practice was predominantly insurance at this time, and so I was seeing practically nothing for my work. I wondered whether it was worth bothering at all.

No more Kangaroo Court

Jean's right shoulder had been getting steadily worse for the last couple of years, and neither I nor the orthopedist could do much of anything with it. We had finally been able to get Workers' Comp to acknowledge that the shoulder was their responsibility, since the problem had developed as a consequence of years of crutch and wheelchair use. The orthopedist had decided that the problem was "impingement syndrome," in which condition the supraspinatus tendon, part of the rotator cuff, chafes against the acromion when the patient raises her arm, because the head of the humerus fails to drop as it is supposed to upon elevation of the arm.

So Jean had surgery in October to shave bone spurs off the acromion, the part of the shoulder blade to which the clavicle is attached. The surgeon determined at this time that the rotator cuff was not torn, as we had feared. He also decided to take a half-inch off the end of the clavicle. Ten days after that, she had an appointment with the IME from her Workers' Comp carrier, who, she told me, did express some puzzlement as to why she was having an IME exam so soon after surgery. Nevertheless, as befits a hired gun from the insurance carrier, writing one of the usual shoddy reports, he decreed that she needed only four treatments a month. We of course needed to protest this. I wrote a letter to the carrier, which they ignored, as usual.

I told Jean that I was not willing to subject myself to an arbitration proceeding (referred to previously as Kangaroo Court). There was one other alternative, which was for her to write a letter to the Comp Board to ask for a priority hearing. She did this. The lawyer's fee for it, $250, was taken out of her check. In spite of that, the upshot of the hearing was that nothing could be decided at it.

After the surgery, Jean had a great deal of pain in the arm and did not get her strength back,as she should have. The problem was not so much where the bone spurs had been shaved off the acromion, as where the half-inch had been cut off the end of the clavicle. It was several weeks before I dared touch this spot, but when I finally could, I found immediately what the problem was.

There was an energetic gap, or interrupted quality between the end of the clavicle and the acromion. Therefore, there was no communication between the clavicle and the acromion to tell the scapula when it needed to move, so I worked to reestablish this. It felt as though I might have been taking the energetic pattern for the correct function from myself and transferring it to her. I had experienced precisely this type of energetic gap in her knees during the first year Jean and I worked together.

Taking care of me

So I was working and getting good results, but not getting paid commensurately, and I couldn't get started writing. I was not sleeping well, either, staying up much too late playing Freecell on the computer. This had to stop. Bleeding and cramping were becoming more frequent again.

The low-grade depression, which had manifested as an un-characteristic lack of interest in food, vanished after I had taken the supplements intended to help deal with poor digestion and candidiasis. Therefore, I am inclined to believe that the depres-sion was largely digestive and fungal in origin.

The A.R.E. had a Health Symposium scheduled for mid-September, and I got a message that I ought to go, never having been to one. Drs. Gladys McGarey and Bernie Siegel were to be keynote speakers. The day I had been intending to leave I spent the entire day organizing the office, a job that had never been completed since I moved in. I learned long ago that if I feel inspired to do a project like that and I have the time, I had better ride with it, since I don't know when the opportunity will arise again.

I had the Lymph Cleanse done on Wednesday so that I would be rested by Friday, when the conference started. Unfortunately, I didn't connect with Belinda the psychic.

The Health Symposium was a breath of fresh air, especially in comparison to some of the Continuing Education programs required by New York State to keep up my license. I found the A.R.E. program much more in tune with my practice and my needs. The presenters were talking about people and energy, not about meeting the needs of insurance companies.

I signed up for a series of teleconferences with Dr. Gladys McGarey and a seminar to take place in May in Austin, Texas. It seems to me there is no one better to learn from than an elder stateswoman of the holistic health movement who also has done pioneering work with the Cayce material.

Besides, I would be doing something for *me.*

On the way home from Virginia Beach I stayed a night at the Rittenhouse, then stopped at Assateague and spent the day at the beach. The mid-September weather was perfect—not too hot, yet the water was warm, having retained a fair amount of summer heat. I sat in the water; when I tried to stand up, the waves knocked me over, so eventually I didn't bother any more. Ponies were wandering around the island minding their own business and ignoring the tourists, as they do. I had extraordinarily vivid dreams that night, which I think were related to the invigorating electrical characteristics of the sea water. The following day I had lunch at the beach at Cape May, extending the vacation feeling as long as I could.

Welcoming the bearer of sleep

I returned to a neat and organized office and began writing. I was still staying up too late, but at least I was accomplishing something.

I went through the bottle of Malic Acid, but didn't see that it was making much difference. Then I ordered the products from Standard Process and watched for my response. I found that the low-grade depression was lifting. A group of us went to a talk by herbalist Kate Gilday at Jean's Greens in October on Ayurveda. She suggested putting ashwagandha in warm milk. Dr. Richard and Karilee Shames, presenters at the A.R.E., had mentioned ashwagandha for adrenals; I had raw milk from the farm and so added warm milk and ashwagandha to my regime at night to aid sleep. The botanical name for ashwagandha is *Withania somnifera. Somnifera* in Latin means "bearer of sleep." That's how I know when to take it!

Adding ashwagandha to the regime seemed to be taking care of the insomnia—in fact, I was sleeping rather a lot. So the body must have been doing something—we would see what it was doing when it came time for the next ultrasound in December. I found I was accomplishing projects around the house, despite feeling sleepy much of the time. Messages in my dreams at this time were about rest. I also increased the castor oil packs again. Castor oil was also helpful topically on my right wrist and ankle.

It was again time to take a look at what I had been getting stuck behind. One answer was the HIPAA Privacy Policy, a federally mandated document that I should have written and distributed in 2003, but ended up having cancer instead. Another was making up the new fee schedule, also long overdue. Another was the computer, which had been without an A drive for quite some time. I had hooked up a replacement, but couldn't get the computer to recognize it, and dial-up Internet was so slow that I wasn't bothering with it at all. I had signed up for DSL in September, but hadn't had it hooked up. In order to do any commodities trading, I have to use the Internet, much as I'd rather not.

So I bit the bullet and wrote and distributed the Privacy Policy and a new fee schedule, and hired someone to straighten out the computer. This accomplished what I meant it to, breaking up the logjam of projects not getting done because the computer wasn't working well.

That fall, a period of enforced rest also served as a time for studying and understanding feng shui on a deeper level. I am not a housekeeper and don't clean for the sake of cleaning any more. Instead, I decide what is annoying me the most or getting in my way and rectify it. If it means changing only one thing, I will still feel the difference.

Twenty-five

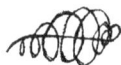

The Need for Rest

Winter 2006-2007

G etting the computer fixed was certainly no guarantee of getting unstuck behind the logjam of unfinished projects; in fact, it broke down again. So did this mean that I had nothing to say, or that I wasn't supposed to say it, or that working on the computer was bad for me (which it is, due to overstimulation from the electromagnetic field it puts out)? After a period of relative rest and catching up on feng shui, the practice got busier again. I got behind, and I found out what "adrenal support" means with regard to ashwagandha. Something that gives "adrenal support" can either stimulate one or knock one out, eliminating the energy needed to burn the candle at both ends. So what was the universe saying now? No computer meant no Internet and another interruption of e-mail correspondence. I went to visit Joy on Cape Cod over Christmas and took the opportunity to warn at least some people that I had fallen into cybersilence once more.

Sometime in late November or early December I had a session with Jenny the acupuncturist, which had become a rarer occurrence, as her schedule and mine got busier. I told her that I was going through some more episodes of bleeding and cramping, and she asked me how old I was. "Fifty-eight," I replied. She observed that my uterus should be going to sleep by now—"But she's afraid to." I communicated with my uterus after Jenny had left and she said she was staying awake to protect me. I can't dispute her logic—if I start overdoing it again, she steps in with the cramps and the bleeding and forces me to slow down.

I came down with a head cold, had the scheduled ultrasound and a Japanese lunch and went home to bed. I always found, while living in New York, that I wanted Japanese food if I was catching a cold. Now I understand the reasons—the high iodine content and this cuisine's tendency to cut through mucus.

I would know by the middle of the next week what the ultrasound had to say. With the ambiguity of last year and the recent increase in bleeding and cramping, I was not sure what it would show this time.

Twenty-six

"Central uterine mass is necrosing"

January 2007

**This piece is rather technical in nature, so you
may wish to skip it. If so, I will summarize it here.**

F ollowing are four ultrasound reports, from studies performed
in April 2004, December 2004, December 2005, and January
2007, interpreted by three different radiologists. The first one read,
"...consistent with invasive carcinoma." The second one showed a
decrease in the size of the uterus. If the cancer were getting worse,
the uterus would be expected to get bigger. But it didn't, so I
figured I had reversed the cancer. The third ultrasound showed a
mass in the middle, bigger than in the second one. The fourth
ultrasound showed the mass getting smaller and dying off in the
middle. Different radiologists disagreed as to the size of the mass.

Whenever analyzing reports for imaging studies, there is always a subjective component that has to be taken into account. So
it is best to use an imaging study as an indicator only, correlated

with whatever is going on clinically. I realized that I kept feeling better, and the AMAS was consistently normal from April 2004 on, so I didn't worry about it very much. However, when the third ultrasound came back showing the larger mass, I decided to increase the castor oil packs to induce bleeding and bring it down again. The fourth ultrasound, with the mass decreasing in size and dying off in the middle, indicated to me that I was succeeding.

A startling utrasound

Sharon Hospital sent the bill so that it arrived before the fourth ultrasound report. I considered this exceedingly rude. Dr. Abby sent me a copy of the report.

I was startled once again by the content of the report. Reading these reports is an exercise in ascertaining inter-examiner reliability. The first two ultrasound studies were read by the same radiologist. The last two were read by different radiologists. The central uterine mass that was necrosing (dying off—this is a Good Thing) was said by this radiologist to be decreased in size from 8 mm. to 6.5 mm (3.15" to 2.56"). The previous radiologist had said that it was 4mm, but it was read by this radiologist as 8 mm. This radiologist made no mention of the thin rim of normal-appearing myometrium surrounding it that was observed last time. The simple cyst on the left ovary, not mentioned last time, reappeared in the report. I suspect it hadn't gone anywhere but simply wasn't mentioned. Overall uterine size was slightly larger. If the thin rim of myometrium had gotten any thicker, as I think it might have done, I would expect this. But the thin rim of myometrium wasn't mentioned this time.

These inconsistencies in radiology reports can drive you nuts if you let them, so sometimes it's a good idea not to take them too seriously. Generally it is a good idea to correlate test results with the current clinical situation, or "go by the cat," as my vet used to say.

To recapitulate the four reports:

1. April 2004: ..."an abnormal appearance of the uterus with marked heterogeneous echo texture in the central portion of it and poor delineation of the endometrial cavity from the myometrium. The findings suggest invasive endometrial carcinoma. No gross parametrial extension [any evidence of abnormal tissue beyond the uterus] although I would suggest further evaluation with CT or MRI [I didn't.] The uterus measures 9.8 x 5.3 x 5.0 cm. [3.86"x2.09"x 1.97"]. Ovaries normal; follicular cyst mentioned on the left one; no ascites [accumulation of fluid resulting from liver failure]. A screening evaluation of the kidneys fails to demonstrate hydronephrosis [excess water dilating the kidney or cystic kidney] although incidental note is made of a possible parapelvic cyst on the lower pole of the left kidney." That was never mentioned again. (Dr. Abby explained that the follicular cyst indicates the ovary is still functioning.) *Radiologist #1*

2. December 2004: "Both ovaries are normal. The left ovary...contains a simple cyst. No ascites. Uterus has decreased in size. It (uterus) measures 5.9 x 5.9 x 8.0 cm. I again a difference date (*sic*) the endometrium from the myometrium. No discrete masses seen. Decreasing size of the uterus although poor delineation of the endometrium from the myometrium is again noted." *Radiologist #1*

3. December 2005: "...compared to a prior study done December 2004. The uterus contains a diffusely heterogeneous mass around which there is a very thin rim of

normal-appearing myometrium. The diameter of this mass is 4 cm. Both ovaries are normal. There is no free fluid. The uterus overall measures 8.6 x 5.2 x 5.9 cm. The endometrial mass appears to have increased somewhat in size when compared to the previous exam." *Radiologist #2.*

Radiologist #1 reported "No discrete masses seen" on the previous exam. Were there, or weren't there?

4. January 2007: "...shows the previously noted large central uterine mass measures slightly less than before (6.5 cm vs. 8 cm. then.) But has a large area of liquifying necrosis within its center. The left ovary...contains a 1 cm simple cyst. The right ovary measures 2 cm and is unremarkable. Overall the uterus measures 9.1 x 6.2 x 6.9 cm." *Radiologist #3*

Boosting the immune system

Radiologist #2 reported the mass as being 4 cm on the previous study; Radiologist #3 reports the same mass on the same study as 8 cm. Which was it? What happened to the thin rim of normal-appearing myometrium? Was it still there? Was it bigger? (This is what I expect.) Was it smaller? If the mass was smaller, but the uterus was bigger, what was the composition of the remainder?

So there you have it. I decided that the liquefying necrosis was a Good Thing. This inspired me to muscle test for the chaste tree berries again and find out if it was time to induce another bleed. Apparently it was. I had been feeling rotten and bleeding during a good portion of the fall. The day of the ultrasound I came down with what turned out to be a nasty cold.

So I guess John Cartmell, the nutritionist with whom I had had some phone conversations in response to the letter I wrote to *The Townsend Letter* that had appeared in the November 2006 issue, was right, and it would be a good idea to boost the immune system—my system was depleted from all this purging. I increased the carrot juice again and started doing castor oil packs almost daily. I could feel my spine becoming looser. I made up some reishi mushroom broth in the crockpot and experimented with different things to add to it. Dandy Blend, the dandelion coffee substitute, works best; the bitter taste of the reishi mushroom broth makes it taste like espresso—well, almost. My morning scrambled egg these days contained chaste tree berries, garlic, dulse, collards, or spinach, maybe a little nettle and astragalus—and the egg, by the way. I soaked the chaste tree berries after having cracked that tooth on one.

My energy was improving after the cold. It took a while, a little over two weeks. I had a busy week and got through it fairly well.

Some days were better. Some were worse. I kept fine-tuning the protocol.

Twenty-seven

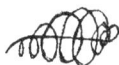

Dr. Gladys McGarey: Living Medicine

Spring 2007

E arly February brought me the first of holistic medicine pioneer Dr. Gladys McGarey's weekly teleconference series, for which I had signed up in Virginia Beach the previous September. She began the series with a brief autobiography, in which she emphasized her medical training during World War II, her life-changing and lifelong interest in and work with the Edgar Cayce material, and the early meetings and discussions with colleagues that led to the founding of the American Holistic Medical Association. The theme of the series was "Living Medicine." Dr. Gladys had become aware of conventional Western medicine as a "War Machine," and I was struck by what she described as the influence of World War II in its formation and development. She spoke of the "kill," "destroy," and "battle" terminology and mentality that now pervades Western medicine as having arisen at this time, and made it clear that she seeks to replace "Killing Medicine" with "Living Medicine."

What a breath of fresh air!

So what differentiates "killing" from "living" medicine? Some of the elements may be the same, but the difference is in the way they are used. Dr. Gladys commented that the *Physician's Desk Reference*, a comprehensive listing of prescription drugs, was only one-inch thick in 1955, while it is at least three times that size now. This represents an increase in the armamentarium against disease, considered the enemy, because "The more you fight, the more you fight." The "kill" and "destroy" attitude toward disease can lead to the disregard and often outright abuse of the person who has the disease. Edgar Cayce's emphasis, on the other hand, was always on the whole person—mind, body and spirit— and his prescriptions usually included some reference to the patient's mental attitude and/or spiritual path. Dr. Gladys also reminded us of the need for the "physician within" the doctor to contact the "physician within" the patient. She left us after that first session with an assignment: "Come to your own conclusions as to why medicine is broken."

Early medicine's feminine face

How did it get that way? Early traditional medicine had a feminine face. Many herbalists and healers were women. With the supplanting of the Goddess and nature religions by Christianity in the West came a shift in the way in which the medicine of the day was practiced. This reached a peak during the Inquisition, when women became suspect, and paganism, rather than being the nature-based religion of country people, began to be considered "evil." In order for there to be an Inquisition, there had to be an enemy.

At the beginning of the twentieth century, there were a number of different movements in medicine, with differing philosophies operating alongside each other, if not in total harmony, at least collegial enough to allow the potential patient something in the way of treatment choice. There were the Eclectics, the Thompsonians, the homeopaths, the osteopaths, the chiropractors, the herbalists, the midwives—and the nascent allopathic movement. The allopaths embraced "science" and decided in 1911, with the Flexner Report, that allopathic medicine was "science" and other methods were not. Science, according to Dr. Gladys, became God. Hospitals became temples and doctors became the high priests. After all, there is ritual in surgery.

Stamping out competition

I see the Flexner Report as a largely successful attempt to stamp out competing types of medicine. (The AMA later formed a "Committee on Quackery" to attempt to stamp out chiropractic. Four chiropractors brought a suit against the AMA for restraint of trade and won it very recently, in 1987. Not long ago, the AMA, a trade organization, created a Scope of Practice committee to "study" the scope of practice of the other professions. A resolution was recently proposed to limit the use of the title "Doctor" in a medical context to MDs, DOs and dentists. It was not passed, because someone realized that only the degree-granting institution that confers the title "Doctor" has the right to regulate its use.)

So if Science=God, and the doctor is a high priest, the patient hands his or her power over to the godlike physician. There are two problems with this: The ultimate healing power resides within the patient, not within the doctor, and medicine at its best is, to my way of thinking, much less than 50% science. Let's say, for the sake of argument, it's no more than 30%. Dr. Gladys makes the distinction that medicine is an art, while science is a tool. For one thing, if medicine were totally scientific, the personality of the doctor would be irrelevant, while nothing is further from the truth. One gets trained in science, but develops the art of medicine.

In chiropractic today, there is a movement afoot to create "Best Practices" guidelines, based on research and science. While, on the surface this seems like a good idea, I have a couple of objections. One is that "science" these days tends to be tainted by the interests of those who are paying for it. I wonder if pure science exists any more.

"Best Practices?"

Another objection is that our invoking of "science" leaves an opening for insurers and allopaths to come up with a latter-day "Flexner Report" and twist it for their own ends. I see the development of "Best Practices" as an attempt to gain respect from the allopaths and payment from the insurance industry and to create some form of "standardization," not necessarily to improve the level of patient care. The trouble is that chiropractic utilizes a wide variety of techniques and methodologies, and is therefore much more difficult to standardize than dosages of antibiotics or pain pills.

These "Best Practices" are being developed by a committee within the profession, but the committee does not necessarily represent a cross-section of the profession. I see a potential danger in imposing "Best Practices," in that they could be used punitively against any practitioner who doesn't conform. There is a similar controversy going on now in allopathic medicine about the treatment of Lyme disease, resulting in proceedings to revoke the licenses of "Lyme-literate physicians" who do not adhere to a certain set of "guidelines."

There is currently discussion in the profession as to whether chiropractic should limit itself to neuromusculoskeletal conditions only. According to the founding principles of chiropractic, adjusting of the spine influences nervous and visceral function throughout the body. This is quite clear from an anatomical standpoint, because the sympathetic chain runs parallel to the thoracic and lumbar spine. So, limiting practice to "neuromusculoskeletal conditions" is actually not a limitation at all. However, insurers and allopaths tend to deny this connection and regard the chiropractic scope of practice not as neuromusculoskeletal, but as musculoskeletal only.

The more external regulation and input from insurers and legislators there is, the more restricted the scope of practice becomes. Before licensure, Doc and his father were successfully treating all manner of conditions that are now considered "beyond our scope of practice."

Yet, studies are still being produced to prove the effectiveness of chiropractic for low back pain. Hasn't that been proven long since? Many of us need merely ask our patients the answer to that question.

"Guidelines" could also be used to deny payment by insurers. The rationale for "Best Practices" seeks to establish uniformity and standardization. The trouble is that people are neither uniform nor standard, chiropractors use a wide variety of techniques and approaches, and similar conditions in different people do not necessarily resolve in the same number of visits. Another problem is that the ICD-9 codes used to define diagnos-

es for insurance purposes are the property of the AMA and
therefore reflect an allopathic, not a chiropractic, orientation.

Norman Cousins commented in *Head First* that a scientist
reasons from the general to the particular, whereas a writer
reasons from the particular to the general. Instead of reasoning
as scientists in patient care, let us reason more as writers. Then
treatments will be tailored to individuals instead of to some
mythical average.

A wartime model is anti-woman

May brought a long-awaited trip to Texas, to attend Dr. Gladys
McGarey's workshop and visit my Houston cousin, whose house
is among tall trees. Houston was definitely not what I expected,
with its rain-forest climate. Walking around, I saw how many
plants grew wild outdoors that I grew inside in pots at home. I
listened to Waylon and Willie on the local country station and
realized how many songs there are about Texas in the country
repertoire. (I found, after returning to New York, that I missed
the nonstop Waylon and Willie on the car radio.)

Dr. Gladys's workshop took place at The Crossings in Austin,
a Texan equivalent of the Omega Institute in Rhinebeck, New
York, from which I receive mailings from time to time. There
were about eight or nine of us, all women, mostly from the
Austin area, except for two who had come from New Orleans and
shared tales of Katrina with us over lunch. I was interested,
though not surprised, to see that all of the attendees were
women. From my observations, the current "wartime" medical
model does not serve women well. The workshop was a series of
discussions and guided meditations, co-facilitated by Dr. Gladys
and Shayla Roberts. Shayla Roberts is a musician and motiva-

tional speaker who has also been a patient of Dr. Gladys's for thirty-five years, and who is therefore very familiar with the concept of "The Physician Within."

I sometimes forget how revolutionary Dr. Gladys's work is. It makes so much sense to me that I feel as though I have always known it. It is less a matter of what she says than it is the humanity and compassion that informs everything she does. She trained in medicine during World War II. A lot of advances were made then, and as I mentioned above, that's when the "kill, battle, destroy" mentality that is now so pervasive took hold. Dr. Gladys's "living medicine" viewpoint, which is oriented toward the person and not the disease, is her response.

Dream work wakes you up

During Dr. Gladys's workshop we discussed the importance of dreams, karma as memory, the relationships between the chakras, and the endocrine system.

The Crossings experience with Dr. Gladys was less didactic than the teleseminars, more experiential in nature. She emphasized on several occasions the importance of recording and working with our dreams. She suggested that we keep a notepad next to the bed and record them as soon as possible, before shifting position too much or going to the bathroom, in order to remember them, and told us stories from her practice about her patients solving their medical problems in their dreams.

To show us that we all do receive psychic impressions and to help us learn to trust them, Dr. Gladys and Shayla instructed us to pair off and use the image of a rose in connection with the other person, then share with our partner what we saw. I saw a Peace Rose with a cut stem, yellow with pink tips on the petals, grown slightly beyond the bud stage, but not in full flower yet. I thought it not very original and wondered if I were seeing anything at all, until my partner told me she was about to get married and was very happy, and she wanted some kind of rose for the wedding with pink tips on the petals—"I was thinking of Fire and Ice [white with pink tips], but that isn't quite right."

For me, my partner saw a "a war zone, chopping through weeds; a white rose, almost fully open."

During lunch breaks, we all sat around the table and talked. Sometimes we shared dreams; at other times we talked about other aspects of our lives. One of the women from New Orleans recounted her experiences post-Katrina, telling us how that situation brought her and her neighbors closer together, and how she had put the Reiki symbols around her house for protection. Hers was the only one in the neighborhood with only minor damage, and her neighbors asked her how she did it.

Choices of the unborn and the dying

After lunch, I walked around the trails with one of the women from Austin, who pointed out the bluebonnets next to the path. "Oh, *that's* what bluebonnets are," I said. I had learned a song about them in elementary school, but had never seen one.

Shayla worked with us for a while with the Drama Triangle (victim/persecutor/rescuer) and talked about the higher vibration of this system, in which the victim becomes Problem Solver, the rescuer becomes Nurturer, and the persecutor becomes Structurer. Then we went on to a discussion of conscious birth and conscious dying. Dr. Gladys referred to the "Second Coming" as the awakening of The Physician Within. She quoted Edgar Cayce as saying, "Ovulation is a law of Nature; conception is a law of God," and said that the incoming soul is aware of everything the mother does. She also talked about choosing who is there when we die. I am reminded of the way my mother did that, choosing Thanksgiving Day for her exit from the world and my presence next to her when she passed.

Shayla then suggested we do an outdoor meditation, in which the direction we faced would indicate our choice as to whether the meditation was to be about mind, body, or spirit. Close-up would mean near future or past; distance would mean distant future. I saw rocks, trees, people, and dragonflies nearby. Then there was a wall, with people crossing behind, which indicated to me that there would be a major shift happening in my life in the not too distant future. Behind the wall were a golf cart and a cleaning lady with a mop bucket; I gathered from the latter that the bleeding probably wasn't going to stop in the immediate future and that my detoxification process would continue. I saw trees and buildings, healthy new growth, old dead growth, and new growth coming up from the center. I thought of the most recent ultrasound results, with the area of liquefying necrosis in the center, and figured that it all was as it should be.

Shayla talked about the Four Directions from the standpoint of a combination of the Sun Bear teachings and Eastern and European symbology. East represents the rising sun, the mind, and the element air; South represents the noonday sun, spirit, and the element fire; West represents the setting sun, emotion, and the element water, and North represents the midnight sun, the body, and the element earth. Shayla also talked about the four-part shield from the Sun Bear teachings, with the four colors—yellow, white, black and red— representing the four races.

The area around The Crossings was beautiful in a stark, desert kind of way that is quite a contrast to the lushness and humidity of Houston. I soaked in the pool and the outdoor hot tub, looking across at the sky, before beginning the drive back to Houston.

Twenty-eight

Polly Put the Nettle On

Summer 2007

After a cold and rainy spring, I was getting very eager to see the sun and be out in it. Barrie had suggested picking the nettles, which were just coming up, and cooking them. I saw to my great pleasure that the nettle patch was thriving and decided to make tea from it every day. The body was telling me in no uncertain terms to spend as much time as I could in the sun. Bill at the store said he wasn't sure if he'd be raising any vegetables this year; he had kept me well supplied for the previous two summers. So I planted some mizuna and tatsoi (greens in the mustard family) seeds I had from last year, and in the meanwhile started picking dandelion greens to put in my breakfast egg. And then I thought, what else can I eat in the breakfast egg? There was plenty of garlic mustard, which has the same peppery taste as others of the mustard family, and there were violets, with their mucilaginous texture. A little later in the summer there would be lamb's quarters, which I hadn't really cared for that much in past years but seemed to be really delicious raw this year. And there would be marshmallow, another leaf with a mucilaginous texture, soothing to the gut, if that should happen to be a problem, and there would be plantain, good either for eating or for putting on wounds, if necessary. Plantain grows anywhere the earth has been trampled. Somebody, either deer or woodchuck, had eaten my first leaves of comfrey, as usual.

I planted a pot of peas and picked up some lettuce and parsley starts at the local farm stands. Having noticed that the lettuces didn't do all that well in the garden last year, I decided to put them all in pots, which worked better. Three parsley plants also went in pots; these also did better than the three in the ground.

Calming and centering, once in the pot

I started making a pot of nettle tea every day in the spring. The tea itself has a calming and centering effect, I find. It helps with arthritis, and I have less trouble with urinary frequency during the night when I have been drinking it during the day. But perhaps more important is the connection it gives me with the land and with the nettles themselves. Picking the leaves every morning is a conscious act, making me aware of the health of the plants, the feel of the ground, the temperature of the air. In early August they had flowered and had a lot of bugs, so most of the leaves I picked were small second leaves. Susun Weed talks of the nettles not stinging, or not stinging as much, if you touch them with intention. I didn't really believe this, but found it to be true. The sting seems to be much worse if I brush up against them accidentally. I do wear gloves when I pick them, though.

On July 9, I picked the first of the blackberries (black raspberries? Blackcaps?). I picked the last one on August 1. The ritual is that I pick the nettles and blackberries first (the blackberries don't make it to the house) and then I pick the rest of the breakfast greens. In early August the yard was still feeding me, though the mizuna was just about over. I still ate garlic mustard, which comes back in force everywhere it's been cut, and violet leaves, and one leaf from the marshmallow, parsley, chives, sometimes oregano, sometimes basil, dandelion, and chicory.

The composition of the yard greens varies throughout the season. I paid respect to the burdock, with its late thistle-like purple flowers. I had been in a lovely green trance in the earlier part of the summer, which seemed to be shifting in August. It was a wonderful kind of deep rest.

I was told by my body this year that I needed to spend a lot more time outside than I had in some previous summers. I did so and found my mood better and steadier, which I think is also partly a function of the nettle tea. I felt relatively strong and tolerated the heat better. The bleeding settled down to a pattern—a bleed every 36-48 hours, but the rest of the time no blood at all. It started in the evening every other day, about two pads' worth, and was over by morning if it started early enough.

The best thing to do when a bleed starts is to go to bed and let the body do what she needs to do, uninterrupted. Lately, she has been considerate in doing that for me. Or perhaps I am becoming a little more intelligent in working with her.

One day I went to bed with cramps, being too uncomfortable to move around or sit. Just about the only things to do in this situation are to read or listen to tapes. So I took out Rosita Arvigo's Mayan Uterine Massage tapes from 1997 (it only took ten years). I checked my uterus according to Rosita's instructions, and sure enough, she had dropped. I moved her easily back into place and worked also on my ribs and low back. Subsequent episodes of cramps were easier, and I continued to spot-check the uterus for position. She is maintaining pretty well. I think the Mayan Uterine Massage (now referred to as Maya Abdominal Massage) is a powerful modality, and I may look into studying it.

Feng shui brings more business

The universe sent several new patients, once I cleaned out the file drawer, some with more interesting and complex problems than the usual. Herbs and supplements were also moving out, since I decided to clear out some of the old ones. Things turned up in the ongoing feng shui process, including the Lyme screening questionnaires from the never-completed Lyme project. Lyme began rearing its head again, and I could at least use the questionnaires for patient files and see if they helped. I thought it might be time to resume the Lyme project.

It seemed I was seeing cancer everywhere. I heard about two friends being diagnosed in a little over a week. I found it frustrating to try to communicate my experience against the powerful propaganda of the medical establishment. It was unsettling. I did not have the faith that their doctors would truly do the best for them, or, more important, know how.

In mid-August I drove up to Nova Scotia, stopping on the way in Sandwich on Cape Cod to meet Joy for supper, and driving up through Boston and up the Maine coast, which I had not done in several years. It was reassuring to see the new green roof on the schoolhouse and to know that it wasn't going to leak and that the floor wasn't collapsing any more. I found a second-hand furniture store in Pictou and got a little computer desk and a microwave. I don't cook food in the microwave, but bought it to heat up hot packs so that the castor oil pack routine would continue uninterrupted. I had also brought along some dried nettles, so I could continue that part of the routine, and noticed much less urinary frequency and urgency since giving up black tea. I missed black tea the most on cold, damp days and gave in to the urge once or twice. Unfortunately I forgot to bring the hot pack with me, but used a cold castor oil pack every night anyway. This was the first year I had brought the laptop to the schoolhouse and I planned to get a bit of writing done. Actually I spent more time making the place more comfortable so I could prepare to write, but that was OK, too.

The grass, non-existent the year before, due to the foundation work, had grown up again. I marveled at the swiftness and completeness with which Mother Nature had made the repair to the land, and I, armed with Rosemary Gladstar's herbal home study course and a field guide, got busy identifying the herbs growing in the yard. Some were the same and some different from the ones I was eating as breakfast herbs at home. There were the ubiquitous dandelions, but no nettles, and there was a patch of sedum around the large spruce tree my mother had planted about thirty-five years ago. Near the outhouse in the back was St. John's wort. I had wondered if I would recognize it, but the moment I saw it I did not question what it was.

I did work on writing Lesson One of Rosemary's course, but that's about as far as I got. Having promised it to someone, I also started the "Handy Household Hints" piece, a collection of useful tidbits I found helpful in coping with different aspects of the cancer. It was two weeks into August, quite a bit cooler than when I had gone up the year before, so I only got to the beach once. I met up with an old friend whom I had not seen in about twenty-five years and met the new neighbors who had bought

Kit's house. They came over to the schoolhouse for one of my traditional gatherings the night before I left.

Contributors to the bleeds

I was beginning to notice something about the bleeding and cramping: There tended to be an unhappy triad of uterine cramping, low back pain, and gas. Any one of the three could trigger the other two. I continued to find Rosita Arvigo's uterine massage work useful, and I eventually discovered that adjusting the ribs as well was even more effective. The summer of nettle tea was making my spine noticeably more supple, as I discovered while doing stretches at the gym. The rib adjustments were helping the digestion to the point that I have had little to no trouble with the hiatal hernia Doc diagnosed back in 1998. The consistent rib work was loosening up the T8-T9 osteophyte. That is a bone spur in the mid-back, just below the level of the bottom of the shoulder blade, that I saw on my chiropractic school X-rays in 1989. Nerve interference from this location may have been a major contributor to both the hiatal hernia and the low back and uterine trouble I developed later.

Jenny the acupuncturist put me back on the Chinese herbs after I returned from Nova Scotia, and I noticed that the cramping was worse again. So I began muscle testing them and discovered that the body wanted me off Ba Zhen Wan, Red Flower, and Zedo Compound, all within about a week. Actually, this made sense, because the Ba Zhen Wan was for building blood, which was quite a lot better by this time, and the Zedo and Red Flower were for dissolving tangling blood stasis in the lower dan tien. (The lower dan tien in Chinese medicine is the lowest of three power centers, located about an inch below the umbilicus.)

When I stopped and thought about it, I realized there wasn't any tangling blood stasis in the lower dan tien any more. The bleeding was spontaneous and effortless by this time, so what the herbs had been doing was making the uterus push too hard. I started the Herbal Iron again, and my energy during bleeds improved.

I was very fortunate to have been given a condition with symptoms that are easy to track. Shortly after I was diagnosed in December of 2002, Pastor Carl of the Sharon Methodist Church had prayed for this, and I see now how vital it has been. I have learned to observe when the bleeds occur, what brings them on, whether the blood is bright or pale, whether there is a lot of mucus, and from this I can infer their meaning. From this experience I have also learned to trust and understand the wisdom of my own body. I have very little fear of diagnostic tests now.

In retrospect, I am glad August was so very restful. September definitely would not be.

Twenty-nine

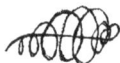

Judith and the
Pitfalls of Chemotherapy

Fall 2007

In order to help my two recently diagnosed friends decide what courses they needed to take, I assembled the written material I thought each of them ought to have and pondered what tack I should take with them—how to voice my concerns so that they would be heard, but not to be overbearing and guilty of the scare tactics used by some in the medical industry. Always mindful of the Al-Anon dictum "not to give advice," I wondered if I might be erring in the other direction.

One of those friends, Judith, told me that in June she had been diagnosed with endometrial cancer by her gynecologist in Panama and sent me a copy of the biopsy report, which was predictably, though unfortunately, in Spanish. The gynecologist had recommended that she be treated in the US. She has a son-in-law who works at Sloan-Kettering, so her son and daughter suggested she go there. Like many people I have known who use alternative medicine for their everyday problems, she did not entirely trust it for coping with cancer.

Sloan-Kettering repeated the biopsy and diagnosed her with papillary serous carcinoma, which they said was far more aggressive than the endometrioid adenocarcinoma I had been diagnosed with. I had visited Judith at her daughter's house in early July and delivered an assortment of teas and writings. It seemed to me that my physical presence was at least as important as the teas and writings, and possibly more so, having experienced at first hand the loneliness of having the world turned upside down. Surgery was scheduled for the following week. After our discussion about lymph nodes, Judith had brought up the subject with her surgeon, who had therefore agreed to take only "sentinel" nodes, minimizing the risks of infection later. If a "sentinel" node is cancer-free, the surgeon figures that the nodes beyond it are cancer-free also and will not biopsy them.

Think twice about chemo

Following up on the mention of herbalist Susun Weed in my material, Judith arranged a consultation with her that turned out to be quite important. Susun, on learning that Judith's blood type was O, told her that she had to eat red meat, preferably something like buffalo. Judith had been a semi-vegetarian for thirty years, eating some chicken and fish, but no red meat, and had a fair amount of soy in her diet. She was hypothyroid. Soy acts as an inhibitor of the thyroid, so Susun Weed advised her to disontinue using it. Susun also advised her to think twice about the chemo or radiation she thought would probably be recommended. Predictably, it was—six chemo treatments with carboplatin and paclitaxel. The doctors at Sloan-Kettering thought she would tolerate it well. I, knowing her better, had my doubts.

She handled the surgery well enough. Chemo treatments, one every three weeks, were scheduled to begin in the middle of August and end just before Thanksgiving, after which she planned to return to Panama. The plan was to take the first two while staying at her daughter's and then stay with a friend an hour north of me for the rest of the time.

It didn't quite work out that way. Three days after the second chemo, I picked Judith up at the train station in Wassaic when she returned from New York City. I had had concerns about the energetics of having someone on chemo staying in my house, but they were dispelled when she told me she had had shooting pains all over her body and decided to discontinue the chemo. "I felt like I was dying," she said.

A healing posture

That was on a Thursday. The following day, Dr. Fran, my chiropractic colleague, was arriving from Chicago for the Chiro Yoga seminar we were attending at Omega over the weekend. I picked her up at the airport and we went directly to Omega, not certain if we were going to make it there in time for supper (we did). This seminar, given by Dr. Steve Weiss, a chiropractor and yoga therapist, would turn out to hold yet another vital piece of my healing process. He described the postures he was demonstrating as being derived from Iyengar and Anusara yoga, and based on ideal posture—the "inner spiral" of the thighs, glutes rotating outward, tailbone scooping down, muscles hugging the bone. I was pleasantly surprised how easily I felt the intent and the result of the posture he described—there was indeed the solidity of the mountain, of everything locking into place.

I have worked with this posture as needed since then, but it hasn't been necessary all that often. I find that since I began doing the Inner Spiral my sacrum doesn't jam the way it used to. (Nerves to the sexual organs come off the sacrum, so releasing the sacrum has quite a bearing on my particular problem.) Adding the Inner Spiral to the Rosita Arvigo uterine massage material made it a lot easier to cope with the bleeds that were still happening every other day.

Yoga, like qigong, puts a great deal of emphasis on the importance of the breath. Because pain is caused by ischemia (not enough blood or oxygen getting to the part), breathing can be used directly as a method of pain relief. I have used the four-part breathing Karen taught us in yoga class on a number of occasions, including when I developed cramps while on an airplane and therefore could not move, directing the breath to the area with the pain. Pain can also result from sluggish lymphatics causing swelling and putting pressure on nerves.

Blood listens when truth is told

I practice frog pose as part of my workout at Curves, not because I like it (I don't), but because I am working to strengthen my knees. It consists of alternately squatting and straightening the legs while keeping the hands on the floor. Frog pose, according to Karen, is particularly good for breast cancer because the up-and-down motion causes pumping of the lymphatics and spinal fluid and aids circulation. Straightening the legs stretches the life (sciatic) nerve, "avoiding shaky legs when you get older." It also raises the kundalini energy from the base of the spine to the top of the head. Karen's definition of kundalini energy is "the best in you."

Dr. Fran flew back to Chicago on Tuesday—the beginning of another workweek, and the weekend, while productive, had scarcely been restful. I felt decidedly overloaded, and also felt that, with Judith, I had been put in a position not entirely of my own choosing, reminding me of the days when I was taking care of my mother, again without having chosen it, or not seeming to have chosen it. And I was mindful of the need not to develop a resentment about that feeling of having no choice.

I am in the middle of a bleed as I write. And I notice, once again, that as I speak truth (unflattering to myself though it may be,) the body says YES! and ebulliently gets rid of another surge of blood and mucus. Could the lesson be any clearer than this? Haven't I been telling patients for years that "everyone needs to tell his or her story"?

Working against chemo brain

Whether I chose to be in this position or not, I was once again being told rather acerbically, "If you don't, who will?" So I tried not to be irritated, though I tend to be during bleeds anyway, realizing that some of the irritation had to do with me, and some of it was triggered by Judith's being weak, and dependent, and forgetful, which wasn't really her fault—she was ill, after all, and had just gone through two rounds of chemo. Another contributing factor to my irritation was the knowledge that the chemo would make it necessary for me to work harder to help her get well, as I would be coping with the toxicity of the chemo as well as the sequelae (consequences) of the cancer.

I recalled a patient of John the acupuncturist in Chicago talking about "chemo brain" and mentioned this to Judith, in hopes that it would reassure her that no, she wasn't going crazy. She had mouth sores for a couple of days as well, and I told her to look up a remedy in Donald Yance's book. There was a formula listing about eight herbs, of which we only had two or three. What finally worked best was simply chewing on a young aloe leaf. She also had a bout of bronchitis, and I put her on reishi mushroom tea to help out the immune system and gave her a Chinese "Clear Air" herb formula. She was concerned that it might develop into pneumonia, but it didn't.

This was a rather trying period for both of us. One afternoon Judith came downstairs teary, depressed, and obsessing about whatever she needed to get done that she didn't have the energy to think about, let alone do. So I made a quick therapeutic decision: "You need burger," I said. And she did. The mood cleared almost instantly. It was easy to recognize this; being a Type O myself, I had been through it, going out for 8-ounce bacon cheeseburgers during the worst of the bleeding.

I put her on castor oil packs, which worked well, and Essiac—which didn't because it gave her diarrhea—and nettle and Goddess tea, and some Chinese herbs. I decided that the rhubarb in the Essiac was the probable cause of the diarrhea; she looked it up on Susun Weed's website and discovered that Susun had a variant without the rhubarb.

The dandy answer to caffeine

For breakfast I fixed Judith my usual one, with Dandy, scrambled egg with yard herbs and dulse, and toast with flax oil, flax seed, and milk thistle seed (for the liver). I figured that her liver had to be quite compromised by the chemo.

Though Judith had brought coffee with her from Panama, we discussed it and decided to use the Dandy instead, especially as she had had some episodes of atrial fibrillation for which she had medication. These ceased almost entirely as soon as she stopped drinking coffee, recurring only if she was under severe stress.

I myself had been introduced to Dandy Blend at the Green Nations herb conference in September 2001. Around that time I had noticed that I had trouble sleeping if I had one cup of coffee at KJ's at lunchtime. Dandelion is good for liver and kidney, and I found it entirely satisfying in the full-bodied way that coffee is, and yet it is also a medicinal. What's not to like? I have also found since then that my patients who use it report very little trouble with caffeine withdrawal—no headaches.

Looking back on it, I wonder how much of the sleep disturbances and late nights on the computer I could have avoided, had I discontinued not only coffee, but black tea as well, a couple of years earlier. As I mentioned, I have observed that black tea can cause urinary frequency at night and bladder irritation, as well as an increased edginess at night. I wouldn't be surprised if the bladder irritation contributed to the cramps as well, by putting additional pressure on the uterus. Because I had been detoxing for several years by this time, I had also become much more sensitive to caffeine, so it now took a much smaller amount to keep me awake at night or to make my nervous system feel jangled.

We also discussed how we would go about testing, and I recommended that she see Dr. Abby in order to check on how she was healing from the surgery and get prescriptions for the bloodwork. I thought the AMAS and the Health Equations analysis would be a good idea. Our research indicated that the AMA titer should drop off sharply between Day 90 and Day 97 post-surgery, which didn't give us a lot of leeway for getting it done before Judith returned to Panama. It couldn't be done until late October. We had the draw done for the Health Equations analysis, but one of Dr. Lynne August's office staffers who handled the data entry was on vacation, so we were a week later than we expected in getting that, and then I had trouble scheduling an appointment with Lynne to discuss it. I suspect Mercury was in retrograde at the time.

Solving the protein mystery

I scheduled my trip to Newfoundland for the week of October 20-28, this being about the latest I could do it. After my return, I consulted with Lynne. She commented on Judith's extremely low total protein and globulin levels and asked me if I thought the chemo was responsible. I mentioned that Judith had been vegetarian for years. Might that be the reason? Good question, Lynne said, and did I have any pre-op bloodwork?

It turned out that the prior bloodwork was post-op but pre-chemo. Albumin and globulin levels had both dropped—therefore the chemo was the culprit. According to Donald Yance in *Herbal Medicine, Healing and Cancer,* carboplatin, one of the two chemo agents that had been used, blocks the reproduction of cancer cell DNA during cell division and paclitaxel, the other one, causes cancer cells to die by preventing the production of proteins and nucleic acids that are required by cancer cells to form DNA. In fact, the production of proteins and nucleic acids is required by all cells, particularly fast-growing ones. So that was what happened to the protein. The components of total protein in bloodwork are albumin and globulin. The globulins are immune system proteins. I also noticed that Judith's cholesterol level went down about 30 points and triglycerides were cut in half. The lowered cholesterol level indicated to me some impairment of liver function, resulting in interference with the making of cholesterol.

No wonder she needed burger so often!

The other major concern on the Health Equations analysis was the elevated Toxin Load score, indicating that the liver was severely burdened. Digestion score was also low. Lynne suggested a number of products containing beetroot to aid the liver, Protefood to increase protein, and Betaine HCl to help the digestion along. I moderated these as best I could to fit within Judith's budget and to keep her from being overwhelmed by a huge number of pills. It was a challenge—particularly as we had already muscle-tested her for the Chinese herbs as well, which her body seemed to want.

After I returned from Newfoundland, we both went to the local hospital to have blood drawn for the AMAS. Judith went in first. The phlebotomist didn't read the instructions and did the draw with a butterfly, a narrow-gauge needle with "wings" on either side so that it can be taped to the skin, and plastic tubing attached. The plastic tubing on the butterfly absorbs antibody, which according to Oncolab lowers the Anti-Malignin Antibody titer by 10-30 points. I caught the mistake, so she did mine correctly, but we had to send away for another test kit to repeat Judith's. Mine was normal again.

Dying from loneliness

I find myself getting tangled in the technical aspects of the story and losing the threads of the more important issue. When she arrived, Judith was not in danger of dying of papillary serous carcinoma or even from the effects of carboplatin and paclitaxel. We would be able to work on those. When she arrived at my house in early September, Judith was in danger of dying from loneliness.

To date I have not found an exception to the rule that there are always emotional issues that culminate in a cancer diagnosis. I recall Belinda the psychic's remark that "Uterus is the mother." I had had relationship problems with my mother; Judith was having them with her children. We talked about the importance of letting them know that, according to Dr. Abby, the risk of recurrence of the cancer was extremely low, and that therefore she was not committing suicide by refusing to continue the chemo.

I had left a book in the room where Judith was staying on the third floor, where I had stayed while I was at my sickest and was doing the same kind of work that she needed to do then. Called *How to Forgive When You Can't Forget,* by Rabbi Richard Klein, it was one of several books that Jean had passed on to me when she was doing her own work. It spoke to Judith and helped her begin by writing three pages a day. I had found myself that writing was a very powerful way of sorting out tangled and chaotic emotions.

But the most important resource we had was our community of friends and neighbors who took Judith in as one of their own. I took her along to yoga class, where she connected up with Dona, who did an Enneagram session in exchange for Judith's writing a newspaper article about her. She joined us at our high-level luncheon conferences at KJ's and went to Dorothy's Mabon ritual. ("Chemotherapy is a lie," she said to us there.) She made friends with my neighbor Patrick, who helped her out with the various complex things she was trying to do on the Internet (not my area of expertise). I watched and admired her ability to find the means and the people to accomplish a wide variety of things.

When one step seems not enough

It seemed that what Judith missed the most in Panama was just such a community of friends. Having been there only three years, she hadn't established such a community yet, and was trying to get a house built despite a difficult contractor and serious cost overruns. She had developed arthritis in her right hip joint and was walking with a cane when she arrived. I adjusted it a couple of times, which helped. One day the pain was so severe that a houseguest offered to do Reiki on it. Later that day I suggested that Judith increase her protein intake at night, an answer so simple and obvious that I had totally missed it. That night she slept well without melatonin and Tylenol and had no pain.

"The eye of the master does more work than both his hands."—From a fortune cookie I once received.

I recalled having shared one of Judith's greatest difficulties, the tendency to think too far ahead. She was trying figuratively to run when she couldn't yet walk. I kept saying, "One step at a time." She was experiencing the same trouble I had had with groundlessness and ambiguity—but that's the way it is, and one gets used to it after a while. It is rehearsing dying, as the Buddhists say. I had ultimately decided to go on living in the absence of any evidence that I was dying, since it seemed to be taking rather a long time and I needed something else to do. I told Judith that the worst time for me had been about six months after diagnosis, before I could quite tell that the therapies were working.

"It's a fierce path you've chosen," she said. " I don't know how many other women would put up with bleeding for seven years." I had sometimes wondered about that myself. Who besides me would be fool enough to take this on? Then I reminded myself that, if I had had the usual hysterectomy, I would have learned nothing and added nothing to the world's store of knowledge. I would have lost control over my own body. I had seen that happen to Doc, and I had feared it much worse than dying.

But now I think I know the *true* answer. If I had simply done what I was told, I would not have been able to teach Judith or anyone else who came after or given them the chance to improve upon my attempt to heal myself, building upon my experience. The payoff has been tremendous. Cancer is no longer a black box. Like other biological processes, it follows rules. It is the body's statement that something is intolerable, but like fusion in an arthritic joint, it is the worst possible choice, a default response. The body will eagerly choose another, given half a chance.

So far as the bleeding is concerned, it is certainly annoying at times, but it will stop when I have learned the lessons I need from it to help other women handle theirs. That is the bottom line.

Ambiguity in retrograde

Judith's first AMAS showed elevated antibody to malignin. More ambiguity. Mercury in retrograde, probably. So we repeated it two weeks later. Due to the Thanksgiving holiday, I had to call

Oncolab a couple of times to get the results of the repeated test. It was normal. It seems that it may take as long as four months after surgery for the AMA titer to drop. So now we know—I think. I did manage to get the news to Judith in Florida before she took off for Panama.

Her children and grandchildren came up here to visit Judith the Saturday before she left, and they all had a wonderful time. I think they were relieved to see how much better she looked, and her son thanked me for taking care of his mother. After that, I think she was ready to tackle Panama again.

And I could get back to my writing.

Judith e-mailed me from Panama in January to tell me about the strategy her local gynecologist was proposing in order to follow up and monitor her progress. The gynecologist was proposing an exam and Pap smear, which sounded reasonable— but then was also recommending an endoscopy and biopsy, chest X-ray, and colonoscopy, all to rule out the metastasis which, in light of the normal AMAS (the blood test designed to show an immune response to cancer) and lack of potential complications on the surgical and path reports, seemed pretty unlikely. I had suggested the AMAS in the first place, precisely to render further invasive, toxic, expensive, and anxiety-producing diagnostics unnecessary. I answered Judith that I thought these recommen-dations sounded like overkill and forwarded her e-mail on to Dr. Abby along with my response.

The AMAS is not commonly used. Why not? There are two possible reasons: one, that rendering expensive diagnostics unnecessary would severely cut into the profits of doctors and hospitals who own the testing equipment, and two, that many mainstream doctors have never heard of it.

Thirty

Enter Patricia

Winter 2007-2008

I don't usually go to Curves on a Thursday morning, but I did on that particular Thursday in October. Patricia was there, filling out paperwork; she was just starting work there, just as Tonia had told me she would be. We struck up a conversation. "Your reputation precedes you," she said. It was quite clear that we were thinking along the same lines as we talked about our thoughts on the current state of medicine. As I recall, she told me she had a strong feeling that I was writing a book about the cancer and that she was going to edit it.

I didn't argue. I knew she was right.

We both became quite excited at the prospect of what this book could become. This was precisely what I needed to hear at that moment, as I was feeling particularly stuck behind the lackluster state of the practice at that time and wondering if it was ever going to change, or if I was ever going to get anything done on the book.

The universe had spoken. This was the time of the shift I had been anticipating, but had had absolutely no idea how it was supposed to take place. Of course I hadn't known. The next piece of the puzzle had not been in place yet, and now here it was. I had, after all, set the intention of working on the book this winter.

Upon Patricia's suggestion, we began the book by meditating together, calling for help from the spirits, and particularly from Doc. Doc came through to her loud and clear; she was astonished at the strength of the connection. "He says he's almost at peace," she told me. "But he says he doesn't want to lose his edge totally or you won't recognize him." This rang true to me. Doc had never been at peace during his time on earth, and I was gratified to find that he was happier than I had ever known him to be. The syntax was right when she repeated what he said to her, liberally sprinkled with Yiddish expressions. He made a comment through Patricia about being a Borscht Belt comic. I had never told her that he had done some acting when he was younger and was decidedly something of a ham.

On another occasion, Patricia and I were sitting at the table talking, and I said again how puzzled I was that Doc, with his knowledge of the Cayce material, had never used castor oil packs.

"He wanted out," Patricia said.

Bingo. *Got it.*

The most important healing modality of all

As I reflect, I consider castor oil packs to be the single most important modality I have used in healing myself of cancer. If Doc had used castor oil packs, he might have begun to recover in spite of himself. As it was, he was ill, and he had lost his license, and as a result, much of his effectiveness as a healer. Chiropractic had been his life. He stayed around just long enough to make sure he had a legacy through me. He got predictably worse from the radiation, then from the allergic reactions he had to the medications he was given to combat the irritable bowel problem that the radiation had triggered. Then, after having the TURP surgery to relieve the urinary obstruction, he became incontinent, which was not only a tremendous indignity, but also took a huge amount of energy to deal with in his already weakened state. Then he made his exit, thumbing his nose at the medical profession, doing exactly what could be expected, considering the style of treatment they offered. I am his voice now.

"Having a complaint is different than having a voice," he says through Patricia.

Being interested in the herbalist's viewpoint on Facial Diagnosis and how it might be different from what we had learned in Physical Diagnosis class in chiropractic school, I went to a workshop with Alicia given by herbalist Margi Flint in early February. Margi's material is based on a combination of Chinese and Ayurvedic thought. She described the three doshas (vata, pitta, kapha). Toward the end of the class, she used me as an example and shared with us what she saw.

Stiff, irritable, and off the castor oil

"Her ears are full, showing a good constitution," Margi said. "There is a little bit of capillary collapse on one of them. The three doshas are in balance, and the kidneys are in balance, which is very rare with Americans. There is some edema in the hands." I thought it would be helpful to explain to the others in the class that I had been treating myself for cancer. I attribute my kidneys being in balance to the nettle tea. Back in 1994 I had taken a self-test quiz in one of Deepak Chopra's books to determine the balance of the doshas, and had decided that I was predominantly kapha at that time. I attributed the edema to the fact that I had stopped castor oil packs to see if that would reduce the bleeding. Thus far, it hadn't. After being off packs for more than a month, I ultimately found myself being stiff, slightly irritable, and vaguely uncomfortable. I was also beginning to have a little recurrence of athlete's foot and itching over the liver, indicating that I wasn't handling sugar quite as well as usual. Ultimately I decided that I would rather put up with the bleeding than feel arthritic, itchy, and irritated.

The bleeds persisted, sometimes daily, sometimes every other day. This became more problematic and more annoying, I noticed, when I ran out of seaweed; I didn't have the extra bit of reserve energy to cope with it quite as well. I also noticed that the morning scrambled eggs tasted flat without seaweed and that I craved salt more often. I started taking Standard Process Thytrophin; this was the first time I had muscle tested positively for it. Thytrophin is a thyroid extract with the hormone removed (this is an oversimplification, but will do for the purposes of the present discussion).

I began using muscle testing much more extensively this winter. Patricia had lent me Dr. David Hawkins's *Power vs. Force,* in which the author discusses the use of muscle testing as a means of determining the fundamental truth in many arenas, not merely the advisability of taking a particular food or supplement at a given moment in time. I found the concept fascinating. I had become acquainted with muscle testing during chiropractic school, though I never formally studied Applied Kinesiology. I had more or less gotten out of the habit of using it until Doc reminded me. We used the technique of pushing down on an outstretched arm, holding the substance being tested in the other hand, and seeing whether the arm being tested becomes stronger or weaker.

Muscle testing in the cat food aisle

Since Patricia called the spirit of Doc in to help us with the book and with our healing work, I "spontaneously" began using muscle testing when shopping for cat food for Wilhelmina, by holding it to my solar plexus and seeing whether I swayed forward, back, or not at all. She was rather choosy about her food, and my usual success rate when shopping for her tended to be about 33 1/3%. With testing, it approached 90%. This saved me a great deal of money. When Wilhelmina was sick recently, Karen told me she had heard that raw clams were good for cats with kidney failure—"Just reporting," she said. I am allergic to clams, as are all three of my sisters, so I know that any positive response I have to clams does not belong to me. I went to the grocery store and tested fresh clams—yes. Canned clams gave a neutral response. One brand of clam juice gave an unequivocal yes; the other was neutral to negative. If I held the can of clam juice and said I was testing it for Wilhelmina, I got an emphatic yes. If I said I was testing it for myself, I got an equally strong no. I took the clam juice home, and she drank two cans of it in two days. Then she let me know she had had enough of it, and later when I tested her for it, she tested neutral.

Karen told me a variation she uses on this muscle testing routine. "If you're testing for the nervous system, hold the thing you're testing up to the third eye," she said. "If you're testing for the immune system, hold it up to the thymus (the upper chest in the midline). For the digestion, hold it up to the solar plexus. For the endocrine system, hold it against the lower abdomen."

These days, I am inclined to believe that I am getting a hint from Doc when it suddenly occurs to me to do something different when working with a patient or when I suddenly decide to use muscle testing differently than I usually do. I had known about Educational Kinesiology (using muscle testing to answer questions) since Dr. Fran and I used to talk about it in chiropractic school, but I had never used it. The concept is simple: The body does not lie. So long as the consciousness and the will do not confound the results—"Keep your mind clear," Doc used to say—it is possible to use muscle testing as a personal oracle.

So, becoming particularly annoyed with the increased bleeding and having (I thought) gone through most of the possible causes, I decided to ask the body about it.

"Your readers are going to want to hear how you know that you're cancer-free and symptom-free, or they're not going to believe you," Patricia said. I replied that the AMAS had been normal since 2004. Actually, the AMAS has been normal since April 2004, at which time the ultrasound read "consistent with invasive carcinoma." I don't think the medical profession has an explanation for this phenomenon, so I will offer a possibility. There may be a time lag between the antibody response and the actual physical signs of the condition. The AMAS is considered to be most effective as an early indicator of cancer, as manifested by the presence of antimalignin antibody, and probably precedes the macroscopic (physically visible) appearance of a tumor. Therefore, might it not be so that it operates the same way in reverse? Might the antibody titer drop before the tumor disappears? To my knowledge, no one except me has tested this theory, as conventional medicine doesn't have the patience to find out if the uterus is going to heal itself, and cuts it out regardless.

Myself as oracle

So, after that conversation with Patricia, I decided to ask myself a few questions. The bleeding had recently increased, concurrently with an exacerbation of problems with a house I owned. Karen thought that the situation might have some bearing on the bleeding. "House equals womb," she said. In my own house, I had begun hiring a cleaning lady to help with projects in the kitchen, and friends had painted the downstairs bathroom, so there was a great deal of change going on. Barbara had stopped seeing clients in my house as of the beginning of February. Patricia reminded me that I had written somewhere about flooding being related to housecleaning, and I had certainly been doing plenty of both.

I had resumed the castor oil packs two or three times a week, and I certainly felt better after that. The bleeding may have increased slightly as a result, but not that much. But it did seem to me that I was doing an awful lot of laundry, which was getting decidedly tiresome. So I asked the oracle—myself—a few questions to shed light on these issues, in a form requiring a simple yes or no.

"Is the situation in the other house a cause of the bleeding?" Yes.

"Is it a major cause?" Yes.

"Am I cancer-free?" Yes.

"Is the uterus healing?" Yes.

"Does Wilhelmina being sick have anything to do with the bleeding?" No.

I had noticed that, as the issues at the other house were coming to a head, that the bleeding was getting worse.

Karen and Patricia, both Reiki practitioners, got together and decided that they needed to work together to help heal Doc's past, by doing meditation and Distance Reiki. They reported that Doc was very enthusiastic about the project, and they both noted that his wife was "in a healing place," still inaccessible. After the second session, they said she was "stirring."

Patricia called me one day, very upset because one of our friends had said, "There is no doubt that Doc murdered his wife." I asked if she had been communicating with Doc during the last few days, and she said no, not since she heard that statement. I asked her to think about what the quality of guidance was that she had been getting from him, and she said it was always good. This reminded me of the many doubts I had had about Doc in the early days, about how it could affect my reputation to be seen with him, about whether I could trust him to work on me. And I told her about the life-changing, and possibly life-saving, experiences I would have missed had I listened to all of the people who thought he was evil, a murderer. Kathleen and I used to talk about that sometimes: Did he do it? "I don't know," Kathleen would say. And I supposed we never would. Patricia came to a conclusion that we both found satisfactory, that the cause of Doc's wife's death had been, at the most, involuntary manslaughter.

"Think about my evolution and not about the past," Doc said once through Karen.

Karen made another suggestion about the issue with the other house. "If someone owes you, release the debt and bless the person," she said, "and then collect your reward, which will be 1000% of what they owe you. You don't want to become karmically attached to the person or the debt. It is important that no one, two-footed or four-footed, be harmed, and that everyone find a better place to live and be happy."

A vision of liberation

I realized that I had been getting stuck behind the issue of the person in question being able to find a place to live with several animals. Karen, Patricia and other friends offered to do spiritual work to help with the transition.

I liked Karen's plan for liberating myself from the situation, which took me out of a box of my own, and decided to work with it that night. I had rather a lot of fun with it, surrounding the person with light, picturing the person and animals on a farm or other wide-open space where all could run free, and decided to add the affirmation that the other house would be left relatively empty, to minimize the amount of work we would have to do. If affirming a reality I would like to see, why not add everything I could think of? So I also added a prayer for Jean, who had been having trouble with her knees again. In the morning I awoke with a feeling of light and clarity that I had not experienced in a long time. For the purposes of artistic license, I would like to be able to say that the bleeding had stopped as well, but this has not happened yet.

Recently I have been focusing on becoming more open to other people's suggestions and ideas and letting go of the idea that I am always right, which I most certainly am not. I thought I had taken care of this one years ago, during my early days in Al-Anon, but it keeps coming up. Patricia sometimes talks about "allowing people to have their character defects." When someone makes a suggestion, and I notice myself having perhaps a slight moment of indignation, I wonder what character defect I am trying to hold on to, and is it really worth keeping? A friend in my Illinois Al-Anon group used to define character defects as "things I do that get in my own way."

It seems to take the better part of a lifetime to achieve, once again, the Beginner's Mind with which we started out.

Thirty-one

Just Ask: At Play in the Universal Field

Spring 2008

I was having quite a lot of fun with muscle testing and started using it for divination purposes. Karen and I talked about it and agreed that it made the most sense to experiment with it light-heartedly, rather than beginning with questions of any major importance.

One day I was considering putting in a Standard Process order, including a kidney supplement for Wilhelmina and one for a patient with a kidney problem, as well as some for other patients. It occurred to me that I might try asking whether a particular supplement was good for Wilhelmina or for the patient without necessarily having it in my hand, since I didn't have either of those products in stock. I had looked in the catalog, and one supplement was a glandular without added herbs, while the other was the same glandular with some herbs added. I could guess which was better for whom, but I had no firm basis for making the distinction. So I asked which was better for Wilhelmina, and I got a "yes" answer for the straight glandular and "no" for the formula with herbs. I got the opposite response for the patient and therefore ordered both supplements. When the patient came in, I asked him to test them both for himself, and he confirmed my original decision.

Either one of the supplements could have been beneficial for the patient. It was unlikely that either would be harmful. I knew that he needed a lot of nutritional help at that time.

A friend of Patricia's, who was also a former patient of mine, came over to visit her while I was at her house one day. The friend was considering trying a gluten-free diet. She had recently been very anemic and had lost weight, which was not a good idea in her case. We had established in a previous conversation that she was a Blood Type O, and I wondered if she had been getting enough protein in her diet. So I asked my usual question, which is whether she was eating any red meat, and she said sometimes. I asked her if she had muscle tested herself for it, and she said no, because she wasn't sure how accurate it would be. She was concerned that she might be swayed by the outcome she wanted, rather than the truthful one.

"I don't know anything about it," I replied, "so why don't you ask me to test?"

She agreed, and started by asking my body how often she should be eating red meat. We came up with the response that she should have it every other day.

"Is the special diet I'm on now good for me?" I swayed backward. No.

"Will she ever be symptom-free?" Patricia asked. Yes.

"Are my symptoms related to Lyme?" Yes.

"Are they related to mold?" Yes.

"Is there a mold problem in the house?" Yes.

"Is the gluten-free diet a good idea?" I swayed a little back, a little forward. Equivocal. Probably unnecessary.

"I ate a sandwich yesterday, hummus, lettuce, and tomato on spelt bread," she said, "and it gave me an upset stomach."

We decided to go through the ingredients of the sandwich one by one to see if we could narrow down the cause of the trouble.

"Was it the spelt bread?" Yes.

She had been avoiding wheat, because she thought she might be allergic to it. Some people who avoid wheat use spelt instead, but it seemed not to be a good idea in her case. I wonder if she might have developed a sensitivity to spelt by using it too frequently as a wheat substitute.

Increase protein to relieve pain

For quite some time she had been on a special restrictive diet that she had learned about over the Internet. Patricia had been concerned that she was pale and seemed to be losing weight, and we both thought it a distinct possibility that the restrictive diet, aimed at eliminating allergens, might be too restrictive, in her case. I remembered a conversation with Dr.Lynne August about a Blood Test Evaluation, during which Lynne had recommended that we increase protein in the patient's diet to reduce pain.

The friend was joining us for lunch, and Patricia had some bread she was planning to serve. Under most circumstances, she would have simply avoided it, but we decided to test for it.

"Is it OK to have the bread?" Yes.

"Is it OK to have butter on it?" Yes.

"Are you sure?" she asked me. "I've been off bread and butter for a long time."

"Try testing it yourself."

She tested it, got an affirmative answer, and ate the bread and butter with great gusto and an utter lack of digestive trouble. Patricia cooked organic hamburger, and she enjoyed that, too. I did suggest that she retest frequently, as the chemistry and the needs of the body are constantly changing.

"I'm not sure how accurately I can muscle-test," she told me. "Several years ago I had surgery and have a titanium plate in my neck. My osteopath told me that the metal would affect that."

"Let's ask," I suggested. "Is it true that the plate makes muscle testing inaccurate for you?" I swayed back and forth. Equivocal. Probably not.

"Was it true when your osteopath told you that?" Yes.

I find this answer absolutely fascinating! It tells me that the insertion of the titanium plate affected her electrical system, but that she has adapted to it over time.

She shed tears of joy when she left us. She felt hopeful again.

Can Lyme cause autism?

April was a month for conferences. In mid-month, Sharon and I attended a Lyme in Autism conference in New Jersey, highlighting the fact that Lyme infection and/or toxicity can be a cause of autism. Autism can also be aggravated by systemic fungal infections resulting from antibiotic use over months, and sometimes years. Shortly before this, I had read an article in *The Townsend Letter* about the relationship between infection and such neurological diseases as ALS, MS, autism, and Parkinson's, and I recalled Jean's telling me once about a high incidence of ALS in Ancramdale, NY, which is a very small place.

"Why?" I asked.

"The iron mines," she replied.

Such conversations have led me to think that much neurological disease is either infectious or toxic in origin. I am encouraged to see that research is being done along these lines. Dr. James Howenstine wrote in the August/September 2008 *Townsend Letter* about fungal infection as a cause of inflammatory breast cancer, as well.

Two weeks later, Alicia and I attended a Self-Care workshop taught by Lucy Mitchella, a massage therapist and herbalist who is certified in Dr. Rosita Arvigo's Maya Abdominal Massage. This is the same Rosita Arvigo who had recorded that Mayan Uterine Massage tape that I had found so helpful in relieving a severe bout of cramps. Lucy began with a detailed discussion of the ways in which the uterus can become malpositioned, and gave us pictures. I certainly found the pictures helpful—the visual element that had been missing from that tape.

Understanding Doc a decade later

So, ten years later, I had a clear image of what Doc had meant in 1998 when he said my uterus was retroflexed and to the right. In her normal position, the uterus is bent forward and the fundus, the uppermost portion, rests on a shelf in front of her. Because she is suspended in the abdomen by several ligaments and moves a great deal, it is easy for her to become dislodged. Lucy mentioned that hollow and floating organs such as the uterus are considered in Chinese medicine to be particularly vulnerable to injury.

Lucy demonstrated the attachments of the ligaments by choosing one of us to portray the uterus and tying scarves to her in various locations, a very graphic way of demonstrating the ligamentous attachments originally explained in this way by Rosita. Lucy also told us that 85% of women experience a malpositioning of the uterus at some point in their lives. If the uterus falls off her shelf, she may prolapse into the vagina, lean backwards and put pressure on the rectum, or she can put pressure on the bladder, as well as pushing against or pulling on the sacrum and possibly causing impingement on the sacral nerves that control functions of the reproductive organs and the bladder. Nerve impingement will, in turn, cause poor communication between the sexual organs and the pituitary, which is supposed to govern them.

On a couple of occasions, I have had patients with low back pain that did not respond unless I adjusted the uterus. If she remains out of position for a long time, adhesions may form between uterus and rectum or uterus and bladder, and there may be leakage from the bladder or the rectum into the uterus, leading to infection.

What also may happen with a malposition of the uterus is incomplete drainage during periods, leading to accumulation of old blood. This is what my cancer consisted of, because old blood that does not move out when it is supposed to can solidify and form a tumor. I saw what I shed.

When I was working a full schedule with seven patients per day, I spent a great deal of time bent over at biomechanically poor angles, so I suspect my uterus was malpositioned quite frequently, since I was in the habit of spending an average of one hour per patient, sometimes more. Along with the exhaustion, the bending was one factor that led up to my cancer, because it impeded the proper drainage of the uterus.

Why my liver was vibing red

During the workshop, Lucy explained another factor that I had never fully grasped before. In her explanation of the menstrual cycle (I have heard and read this many times, so perhaps my eyes and ears tend to glaze over a bit), she talked about the role of the liver, which produces fibrinogen and antifibrinogen at different points in the cycle. Fibrinogen is produced at the same time as progesterone, in order to create a firm bed in the endometrium to welcome the putative fertilized egg. Then, if the putative fertilized egg does not appear, the liver is supposed to create antifibrinogen to permit the shedding of the endometrium.

But what if the liver is impaired, as mine was four years before I was diagnosed? (Remember that Doc had told me in 1998 that my liver was "vibing red.") Gerson says the liver is always impaired in the case of cancer. The antifibrinogen may not appear on schedule, in time for the menstrual period, so that old blood may accumulate instead of bleeding out as it is supposed to. One thing I noticed while the cancer was active was the peculiar texture of the blood—it was sometimes so viscous that it could almost be rolled into a ball.

Another consequence of poor liver function is inadequate breakdown of estrogen, which, when in excess, will cause the endometrium to keep proliferating. Possible endometrial cancer is often observed on an ultrasound when the endometrium is too thick. Estrogen replacement therapy is, therefore, a risk factor for endometrial cancer.

An amazing anatomy lesson

When Lucy went on to discuss the causes, signs, and symptoms of a malpositioned uterus, I recognized several that I had had at one time or another, and I think all of us in the workshop did. Some causes of a malpositioned uterus seemed self-evident, such as repeated pregnancies with too little time in between to allow the ligaments to heal, or bad professional care during or after pregnancy, but some were less obvious, such as walking on cold, wet grass, which causes muscles to contract and thereby impair circulation. Most of the symptoms of uterine malpositioning were the direct or indirect consequences of poor drainage of the uterus (direct) or of pressure of the uterus on surrounding organs (indirect).

I was quite impressed with the detail of the anatomical review Lucy gave us and found it was better presented than it had been in chiropractic school. It is also possible, however, that I understood it better because of my intervening years of experience.

Lucy then taught us how to do the self-massage. We ran through it twice, and we also had the steps listed on a handout so we could refer to it later. It consisted of pulling up on the uterus toward the navel, from the center, the right and the left, a lymphatic massage working upward in circular motions from the thighs, and then working down the midline from the xyphoid (the point on the lower end of the sternum) and from either side, from under the ribs to the navel. My uterus felt considerably more relaxed after this. It did provoke some additional bleeding, but this was not surprising.

Then she told us to lie down while she played us a meditation for the uterus, narrated by Rosita. We were to note our reactions to the following suggestions:

Remembering the birth process: I felt stiffness and apprehension. Having gone through the GIM work and remembering the strangled child, this made sense.

Being held at mother's breast: No particular reaction.

Menstruation: Tremors.

First menstruation: That was OK. No problem.

Making love: She likes that. Warm and expansive feeling.

Pregnancy: HELL NO!

Labor and delivery: Shaking. I had remembered hemorrhaging to death during childbirth in a past life.

Favorite lover: Don't think I'll share that one here.

Lucy quoted Don Elijio Panti, the Mayan shaman who was Rosita's mentor: "If a woman's uterus is off center, her body, emotions, and spirit are off center."

Think about that.

I was most impressed with this workshop and am considering going on to do the professional training, which is the next level, enabling us to apply this modality in our practices. Beyond that are two levels of certification courses, the first for professionals who wish to be listed as certified practitioners, and the second for those who want to teach.

The body never lies

After the workshop, I was inspired to find out a few more things about the course the cancer took, since I can ask anything I want, so long as the answer can be Yes or No.

Was the cancer gone in April 2004? Neutral; equivocal. At that time, right after the broken leg, the AMAS blood test was normal, but the ultrasound showed "invasive carcinoma."

Was it gone in May 2004? Yes.

Tonia and I had done the parasite cleanse in late April. Was that important? Yes.

Would the cancer have gone, had I not done the parasite cleanse? Weak yes.

Essiac, carrot juice, and acupuncture were all important as well, according to the muscle testing.

Was there a mass in the uterus in December 2004? No. December 2004 was the date of the second ultrasound, in which the size of the uterus had unexpectedly (from a medical standpoint) decreased. Radiologist #1 had made no mention of a mass, but Radiologist #2, in comparing it with the subsequent film a year later, had said that there was one.

Was there a mass in the uterus in December 2005? Yes. Radiologist #2 had described this mass as being 4 cm. in diameter.

Was there any living tissue in the mass? No.

Was it necrotic, dead tissue? Yes.

Is there a mass now? (late April 2008) Yes.

Is it 2 cm.? Yes.

Is there adenomyosis? Yes. Adenomyosis is a condition in which the endometrium eats into the muscle, or myometrium.

Is that a result of the cancer? Yes.

Was the sore (adenomyosis) 3 ½ centimeters at its largest? Yes.

Is it 1 cm. now? Yes.

Is the bleeding more from the sore than the tumor? No.

Is the bleeding more from the tumor than the sore? No. About the same.

Is the uterus healing? Yes.

Is the cancer gone? Yes.

Will the bleeding decrease before it stops? Yes.

Will the bleeding stop when the situation in the other house is resolved? Strong yes.

Will it stop before July? Yes.

About bloodwork: Is the AMAS still normal? Yes.

Is Serum Ferritin at 21? Yes. (Serum Ferritin has to do with the amount of iron the body has in storage. A level of at least 20 is recommended. It was at 16.5 the last time.)

Is Serum Iron higher than last time? No. (Still work to be done on this issue.)

Are Triglycerides about the same? Yes.

Is Serum Insulin over 9? No. (This would be an indicator of diabetes.)

Is it 7? Yes.

Is Fasting Blood Sugar 89? Yes.

Do I have a candida problem now? No.

Did I have one before I took the Zymex 2? Yes.

Is protein about the same? Yes. (Lynne had told me it was a bit low.)

A few weeks have passed since I asked the questions above. The last few chapters of this book are being written in real time, so readers may make discoveries with me and see the changes occur as they happen.

By mid-May, the situation in the other house, while not totally resolved, was moving toward resolution, and I noted in the bleeding the reflection of the different stress levels I was experiencing, according to what was going on at the moment. The bleeding pattern changed again and once again I was having a night with no bleeding alternating with a bleed. So I got curious and asked about the bleeding again.

Is the bleeding related to the tumor? Yes.

Is it related to the adenomyosis? No.

Is the adenomyosis healed? Yes. (I keep rechecking this to make sure.)

Is the tumor 1 cm. now? Yes. (It was 2 cm. a couple of weeks before.)

Jean takes a fall

On the night of Mother's Day, I had been out. Patricia told me she had a feeling I should check the answering machine. There were messages from Jean and Teresa, telling me that Jean had fallen on cement as a consequence of her left knee giving way, and she was in the hospital with a shattered left hip and left wrist. We had been struggling with instability of the left knee for years, a consequence of the patellar tendon being reattached too far to the left when the kneecap was removed. The removal of the kneecap itself also eliminated an important strengthening and stabilizing mechanism of the knee joint. This fall necessitated a hip replacement and repair of the wrist, which turned out to be a more serious problem than the surgeon had originally anticipated.

Teresa started the prayer chain going immediately, and I convened a circle with Karen and Vicki, with remote assists from

Patricia and Teresa. Karen saw a golden mesh down the entire length of the leg and said that the problem had been the leg twisting. Despite my not having talked about the specifics with her, Karen was entirely accurate.

"I saw her in a spirit hospital, with a lot of people rushing around," Karen said. "It was quite clear that she had a lot of people praying for her." She commented further that the injuries on the left side of the body have to do with ancestral patterns, while injuries on the right have to do with past lives. All of the injuries from this incident were on the left.

Vicki visualized rainbow sheets, one color for each of the chakras, to help with the healing. I, following Karen's lead, focused on Jean's mother and reminded her that she owed Jean a big one, and that Jean needed her help now.

Thirty-two

Mapping the Road to Cancer

May 2008

Having decided, under the influence of Doc (in spirit) and Dr. David Hawkins, that I could use muscle testing to ask my body anything I wanted to, I asked a number of questions about the origin and progress of the cancer. Despite having only questions with a "yes" or "no" answer available to me, I have been able to come up with an explanation that satisfies me.

So here's what I discovered:

Between 1995 and 1997, I remained by and large fairly healthy, despite the stresses of starting the practice and living in a moldy environment, because I was still getting outside quite often and doing a lot of walking. My diet then took a turn for the worse because I had inadequate cooking facilities and not much money. Between early 1995 and late 1997 I gained about 25 pounds.

The pathology begins

The year in which the pathological process that eventually turned into cancer really began was 1998. I became hypothyroid that year, due to the mold in the office, which affected me more than before, because I was working more and getting outside less. Late that year I also began having problems digesting pasta, a problem I had never had before, as well as joint pains, which I eventually ascribed to eating too much beef and potatoes. The beef I was eating then was not organically grown, unlike the beef I eat now, and therefore may well have contained hormones. These could have contributed to estrogen dominance. This means that, when there is too high a proportion of estrogen to progesterone, the uterine lining fails to break down completely each month, and there is, therefore, an accumulation of endometrium from month to month.

The role of the liver and of mold

The liver is responsible for breaking down the excess estrogens, and wasn't doing so adequately. The liver has more trouble breaking down foreign estrogens, such as those in plastics or those added to commercially grown beef, than the estrogens the body itself produces. Mold was also contributing to the impaired liver function. Poor liver function also made conversion of thyroid hormone from T4, the storage form, to T3, the active form, less efficient, so there was an interaction between thyroid and liver, creating a vicious circle. I gained an additional 20 pounds in 1998 alone. Dr. Ritchie Shoemaker, in *Mold Warriors,* mentions this type of weight gain as an effect of mold toxicity.

This is what was happening when Doc told me my liver was "vibing red" in late 1998.

Correcting for the liver problem

Doc started me on B complex and digestive enzymes and adjusted me for the hiatal hernia. Muscle testing tells me that there was still a thyroid imbalance after 1998, but I was no longer hypothyroid, because we had cleared up the liver and digestion enough so that conversion from T4 to T3 was more efficient. I still thought that my periods had slowed down more than they should have. Due to Doc's interventions, I was able to increase my patient load. This was not what I should have done.

When I started eating seaweed daily in the spring of 2000, this brought the thyroid back into balance, and my energy increased. The liver was improving in 1999 and 2000. When the bleeding began in September 2000, it was a consequence of better thyroid function and an attempt by the uterus to clean itself out—-an attempt at correction, as I had thought at the time.

My liver function worsened somewhat in 2001, probably due to increased stress, and the adrenals went out of balance then. Though the bleeds were not severe, they were also unresponsive to anything Jenny the acupuncturist and I tried.

Castor oil packs and yeast

I had the first Pap test in January 2002. I had a yeast infection at that time. Although I started castor oil packs immediately after that and they cleared the joint pains, the yeast infection, and a fungus nail I had had since 1995, the yeast infection nevertheless served to trigger the cancer, probably due in part to an increased sensitivity to yeast because of the previous mold exposure.

The second Pap test, done in late March, had the same result as the first. I did not have cancer in March, but by April I did. The flooding began in earnest at the end of March. It had not yet involved the myometrium. The liver imbalance was triggering a kidney imbalance by this time, according to my muscle testing.

Cancer and Lyme

So I had cancer by the time I came down with Lyme, though I didn't know it yet, and my immune system was down, as Dr. Lynne August had said. The fact that the cancer did not affect my healing from Lyme would indicate that my immune system may have been down, but it was not seriously impaired. I was doing castor oil packs daily and huge amounts of Vitamin C and Goddess tea, and the month's worth of doxycycline turned out to be enough to take care of the Lyme. The bleeding backed off somewhat during the Lyme. I became anemic for the first time.

While the cancer did not affect the Lyme, the Lyme affected the cancer by putting further strain on the liver. This in turn created an overbalance of estrogen, because it wasn't being broken down as well as it should have been. The thyroid was still working normally. The cancer had not eaten into the myometrium. I spent the fall recovering from Lyme and not having much energy. When I tried to increase the patient load again, I couldn't.

The diagnosis and what we did about it

So the cancer had been going on for about eight months at the time of diagnosis. It certainly was not progressing rapidly. But the diagnosis told me I had to get more serious about coming up with a protocol. So I started with the Essiac and juicing then, and Jenny the acupuncturist and I did some trial and error before coming up with the right mix of Chinese herbs. The Essiac, Red Flower, and Xiao Yao Wan contributed to the fever I had shortly after diagnosis, by kicking my immune system into gear. By December 2002, the cancer was starting to eat into the myometrium.

I was fatigued and feverish in late winter and into the spring. The smoldering that had shown up in my drawing after the first GIM session in January had become hot reds and yellows in May and into June, before beginning to cool down to blues in later June and early July. In June, the AMAS was borderline. In May, I was rehearsing dying. I might have actually done so if I hadn't decided to stop work over the summer.

The dental connection

The cancer, at its most virulent in July 2003, had begun to reverse in August. During July I had had an emergency root canal done, which ultimately failed and resulted in extraction, but having this source of infection removed, along with three other broken-down amalgam fillings, contributed to the reversal. Estrogen levels were starting to drop as liver function was improving. So my energy was good enough to do the Crop Walk in September, but it wasn't really good enough yet to resume a work schedule. Unfortunately, I had to. This put more stress on the adrenals.

Then my mother died.

Broken leg and enforced rest

In January, I had decided to do the first ultrasound, but the universe decided I wasn't going to, and that I would have two months' enforced rest with a broken leg under Olive's expert care instead. This was a Good Thing. I still had cancer in January. In February and March, it was abating. In April it was almost gone. The AMAS was normal, but the ultrasound was read as being "consistent with invasive carcinoma." While there was still some living tissue in the tumor then, most of it was already necrotic. Perhaps the ultrasound could not differentiate this. I did the parasite cleanse soon after the AMAS and ultrasound. If the cancer had been triggered by yeast, it makes sense that the parasite cleanse would have been helpful.

The cancer was gone in May. So John the acupuncturist in Illinois was right when he said in August that I was doing better than I thought, and that he didn't see cancer anywhere in my field. John had told me to pay attention to the kidneys. Liver function was normalized by this time; kidney function, not quite.

Breaking down the cancer

The heavy bleeding from May until December represented the teardown of the cancer. The peak of the teardown was in October 2004, probably at the time I recall having the last flood. The ultrasound in December 2004 showed a decreased uterine size, reflecting this; the AMAS was still normal. No differentiation between endometrium and myometrium shows on this study. Bleeds continued, no longer hormonal.

The teardown of the cancer caused a 3.5 cm tear in the myometrium, which was the major cause of the bleeding in 2005.

The role of exercise

I began working out at Curves in July, hoping to rehabilitate the broken leg and improve hormone and liver function. Increasing circulation through the liver via exercise would improve its efficiency, so that it would break down estrogens as it was supposed to. I added one of Karen's yoga poses to my routine, one in which I lie on the left side, elevating the right leg, doing Breath of Fire (panting through the nose). This further increases oxygenation and circulation through the liver.

A mass appears on ultrasound

I was taken aback when the December 2005 ultrasound showed a "4 cm mass" where there hadn't been one before; however, now I think I understand it. It is analogous to the time Patricia started taking Xiao Yao Wan, twelve pills a day, and a boil almost immediately appeared under her arm. In my case, because the liver was functioning normally again, it was gathering toxins and eliminating them by the most convenient, established route— from the uterus, through bleeding. The ultrasound no longer called the mass "consistent with invasive carcinoma," and in fact, it wasn't given any label. The mass was entirely dead tissue, according to my information.

In response to that ultrasound, I increased the castor oil packs again, hoping to speed up the removal of the toxins and get rid of the tumor. The bleeds now resulted from a combination of the tear in the myometrium—adenomyosis—and the shedding of the tumor.

The next ultrasound, January 2007, showed the tumor shrinking and with a large area of liquefying necrosis in the middle, so this strategy was working.

The role of Maya Abdominal Massage

In April 2008 I took the Maya Abdominal Massage workshop. Shortly thereafter, I asked through muscle testing about the size of the tumor then (2 cm.) and the size of the adenomyosis tear (1 cm). A couple of weeks later, after having done the self-care routine several times, I received these answers:

The tumor was down to 1 cm. The adenomyosis was healed. The cysts on the left ovary and left kidney were gone.

As of May 28, the tumor was 7 mm. I was told by my muscle testing that the bleeding was to end as of June 4.

Note: The next two pages contain a graphic timeline illustration, visually mapping the road to cancer described in the preceding chapter.

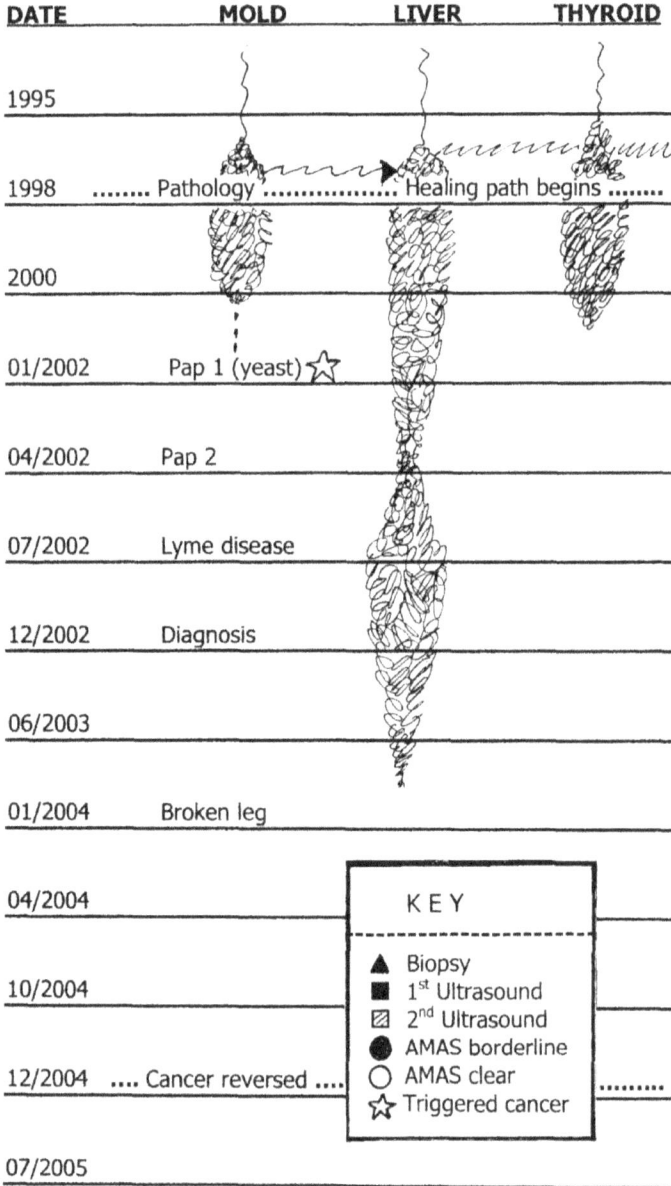

DATE	MOLD	LIVER	THYROID
1995			
1998	.... Pathology .... Healing path begins		
2000			
01/2002	Pap 1 (yeast) ☆		
04/2002	Pap 2		
07/2002	Lyme disease		
12/2002	Diagnosis		
06/2003			
01/2004	Broken leg		
04/2004			
10/2004			
12/2004	.... Cancer reversed		....
07/2005			

KEY

- ▲ Biopsy
- ■ 1st Ultrasound
- ▨ 2nd Ultrasound
- ● AMAS borderline
- ○ AMAS clear
- ☆ Triggered cancer

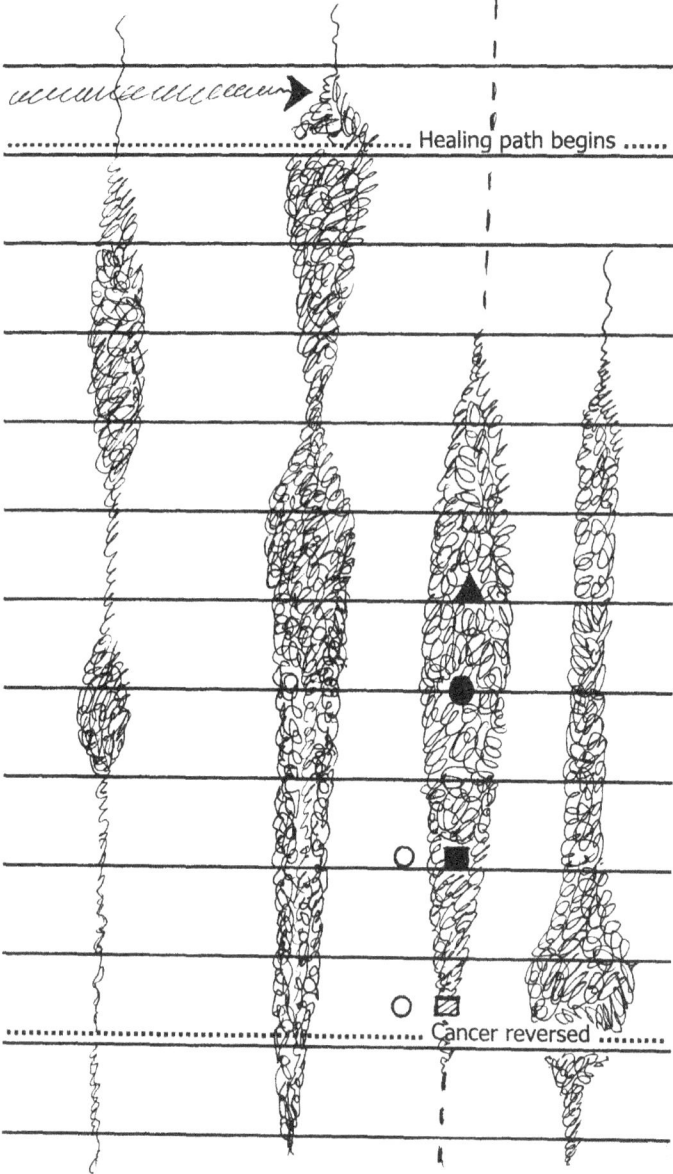

KIDNEY/ADRENALS   ESTROGENS   CANCER   BLEEDS

Healing path begins ......

Cancer reversed ....

Thirty-three

The Bleeds

June-August 2008

The bleeds didn't stop on June 4. The stressful situation that I considered to be a major cause was dragging on, so this wasn't a surprise. (I had already been told through muscle testing that the tumor and the adenomyosis were gone, so were no longer causing them.) As the stressful situation was dragging on, the bleeds seemed to be getting a little worse, and I have to admit I was getting a little fed up with both the situation and the bleeds. What more was I supposed to do? Most important, was my guidance good enough to trust? Or were the results I got through muscle testing being swayed by what I wanted to happen?

So, then, what is the point of the bleeds continuing? Am I not getting some message that I am supposed to get? I've been asking this question and am coming to the conclusion that the bleeds are continuing so that I can extract as much information as possible to pass on to others before they stop—to analyze as many physical, emotional, and spiritual causes as I can.

The bleeds have had different causes and characteristics at different times. During the early days of the cancer, they were still hormonal; later, they were not. During the flooding, there were many chunks and clots; now there are none. Then, the blood was bright or dark; now it is pale and diluted. Sometimes stress would bring them on. At other times, a bleed would occur when the body was happy and relaxed, as in the gong meditation during yoga class or while exercising at Curves. Trying to predict them and second-guess them has not worked out very well most of the time, and perhaps there is a lesson in that, too—it is to trust that my body knows how to heal herself, and to allow that to happen. Sometimes I merely have to get out of the way.

A dramatic attention-getter

The initial purpose of the bleeds was quite clear—to get my attention. On a purely physical level, the purpose was to clear out the excess endometrium that had built up due to the estrogen dominance resulting from impaired thyroid function.

I remember saying in 1999 that the practice was bleeding me to death. Actually, it was the Workers' Comp system at that time that was most disturbing, so I reduced the load of Comp patients. In doing so, I discovered one vulnerability I had—my sense of responsibility for the ones who were in severe pain and needed a lot of treatment and were getting no help from anywhere else. I felt I could not abandon them yet, in simultaneously coping with their illness and fighting a system that was opposing me at every turn, I was exhausting myself more than I was helping them. One failure takes more energy than ten successes.

Karen did a session of the Emotional Freedom Technique with me, and she came up with precisely what I needed to hear:

"Don't waste your energy on the ones who aren't going to get any better," she said.

Bingo. Got it once again. Those are the ones who bleed me, if I allow it. Whether they are patients or people in other contexts who are running themselves on my energy, the principle is the same. I probably need to go to Al-Anon again.

As Judith had said the previous fall, I also had to look at how many women would want to heal their own cancers in this way if it meant putting up with almost eight years of bleeds. I have proven that it is possible to do just that, but would I have wanted to, if I had known what was coming? Or would I have gone for the medical "quick fix" that really isn't one?

I doubt that everyone who heals an endometrial cancer by natural means has to look forward to seven or eight years of bleeds. My friend Sooz, who is also treating her endometrial cancer naturally, tells me that she has had much less of a problem with the bleeds than I have. Indeed, I may have been given this symptom because I would take the time and have the knowledge base to listen to and interpret these messages from my body, rather than choosing to have a hysterectomy, thereby learning nothing. As more women reject the conventional options, we will learn much more about the natural healing process for endometrial cancer. There quite clearly is one.

There are already a few of us natural survivors who are in touch and are sharing our information. One friend, cancer-free for many years, says that she still bleeds when under stress. So the bleeding serves to let her know that she needs to find a better way of coping with the stress. What a gift that is—the cancer has given her a known symptom, annoying but not serious, serving as a warning. It seems to me that the allopaths have a tendency to overreact to uterine bleeding, which can be an attempt of the body to normalize. While it certainly makes sense to find the source of the bleeding and determine the presence or absence of pathology, it isn't always necessary, or even desirable, to stop it.

How many more are out there whose healing I know nothing about?

Another method of nutritional testing

Toward the end of June, Standard Process sponsored a seminar on Nutritional Response Testing, a method of evaluating patients' nutritional needs using muscle testing. Developed by Dr. Freddie Ulan, a chiropractor, this system achieves more specificity by combining use of a full body scan to pinpoint the location of the problem, and test vials containing homeopathic preparations of heavy metals, potential food allergens, infectious substances, and toxic chemicals. The fifth major stressor for which the patient is tested by this method is scars, some of which can be problematic while others are not. Scars are not only those resulting from surgeries or injuries, but also vaccinations, tattoos, piercings, tooth extractions, or acne scars. Nutritional Response also tests for "blocking" and "switching" of the autonomic nervous system, either of which can render good remedies ineffective, due to the resulting inaccuracy of the body's response to a stimulus. "Blocking" is the inability of the autonomics to upregulate or down-regulate to match the current situation. "Switching" is the autonomics' confusion and inconsistency of response. After the area or areas of weakness have been determined, the Standard Process supplements that apply to that problem are muscle-tested for appropriateness and dosage.

I thought this use of muscle testing interesting, and was tested at the end of the seminar by the instructor, Dr. Darren Schmidt. No weakness turned up in the uterus. This confirmed the conclusion I had reached through muscle testing that there is no cancer or other lesion remaining there, and that the bleeds no longer relate to a tumor.

What did turn up was a weakness in the left kidney, the one with the "parapelvic cyst" visualized on ultrasound in 2004. (I had been subsequently told by my body that the cyst was gone.) The digestive weakness that Dr. Lynne August had found previously on the Blood Test Evaluation showed up again, and Dr. Schmidt recommended I take Multizyme for that, an enzyme formulation without acid. This time there was no mention of low stomach acid, as there had been before, so perhaps the nettle tea has been helping me maintain electrolyte balance better, since I haven't been on Lyte Cl electrolyte solution in quite a while. Dr. Schmidt recommended two products for kidney. He also told me that I had a wheat sensitivity, to avoid wheat and be careful with grains in general. I had suspected the wheat sensitivity, but found it quite inconvenient, so was probably ignoring it more than I should have.

Within a couple of days, I noticed results from these interventions. I started the enzyme first, before the other two products arrived in the mail. The remains of my head cold disappeared quite quickly. The day I began the two kidney products, I felt a feeling of expansion in my low back and have had less urinary frequency at night, even when bleeding. Avoiding wheat is more difficult. When I don't, though, I notice nasal congestion and more afternoon sleepiness. One of my sisters also has a wheat sensitivity. The sleepiness could also be sugar-related, as I have noticed it sometimes after having a muffin or other sweet pastry after lunch. So I am doing that less often.

As that troublesome situation with the other house wound down, I kept being told that the bleeding would stop, but it didn't. It did decrease in volume, especially at the outset, and it has by and large resumed its every-other-day pattern. During the most stressful period, the bleeds had become daily occurrences again, and more voluminous, though still much paler and lacking clots than they had been during the flooding. This confirmed my observation that they were a response to that stress.

The bleeds are only the latest of many stress responses I have had over the years, the response I developed because of the cancer. The purpose of a stress response is to get my attention and to force me to change whatever pattern of behavior led to it. Unfortunately, sometimes I am so clever that I figure out how to foil the stress response, so that it no longer serves its purpose. In chiropractic school, the "slow down" message was delivered to me through low back pain. I taught myself "sending" and other ways of working on low back pain, so that didn't work quite so well any more. Lyme disease was another attempt at slowing me down, but I took my doxycycline and any number of other things and got better a little too fast to get the rest I really needed.

The cancer did get my attention, and I hope I got the message this time—except, after my mother died, I really didn't, so I slipped on the ice and broke my leg. That wake-up call was really hard to ignore, and it worked.

It's hard to run around in circles when one's leg is in a cast.

A lesson from Wilhelmina

Other factors have contributed to the continuation of the bleeds. Wilhelmina, the cat, had been diagnosed by the vet with kidney failure some time before, but in the spring the situation became serious enough that she had to be hydrated subcutaneously, either daily or every other day. It therefore became much more problematic to leave her alone, and this became another major stressor.

Kidney failure is a common cause of illness and death in older dogs and cats. The conventional approach is to put the cat or dog on a low-protein diet, in order to reduce the strain on the kidneys. We tried this; it didn't work. My suspicion is that kidney failure in dogs and cats is a disease of civilization and deficiency, like cancer or heart disease in humans, resulting from an unnatural cooked-food diet.

I recalled reading about Dr. Francis Pottenger's cat studies, in which he raised two groups of cats, one eating a diet of only cooked food and pasteurized milk, the other eating raw food and raw milk. The cooked-food cats developed skeletal and reproductive abnormalities and died out by the fourth generation. Dr. Michael Dobbins had alluded to this study in remarking, partially in jest, that he was in "the third generation of Pottenger's cats."

Tong Ren, another healing modality

Patricia and I went with two other friends to a Tong Ren healing session in West Hartford. I had heard of this before and read about it, but never witnessed it. Tong Ren is a system invented by Tom Tam, using elements of acupuncture, chiropractic, qigong, and sound healing. On the first glance, it appears rather bizarre. The healer, Dr. Ming Wu, stands in the front of the room and asks the patient to tell his or her symptoms. In response to that, he calls out a list of acupuncture points and spinal levels and—in this particular case—strikes a large gong in varying patterns, depending on what the complaint is. Each of his students in the room holds an acupuncture doll and a small hammer and strikes the points on the doll with the hammer as he calls them out. This serves to focus the qigong energy on the level where it is needed. He is quite clearly feeling the energy and responding to it, lowering his hands when he feels the healing is done.

Tom Tam originally developed this system to work with cancer patients, and several who attended what Wu calls his "Guinea Pig Class" were under medical treatment for some serious conditions. Some reported improvements, and all seemed to have a feeling of hope. While the treatment may appear odd, it combines elements of several sound and proven modalities. Acupuncture and chiropractic both deal with the electrical energies of the body; acupuncture uses the meridian system of energy pathways associated with the various organs, plotted out by the Chinese five thousand years ago. Chiropractic deals with the influence of the spine on the nervous system, and thereby on the entire body. To all this are added the vibration of the gong and the same collective energy used in healing prayer. One session is quite clearly not enough to get a good sense of how it works, but one of our friends commented that each time she goes, she leaves walking better than when she arrived. At the end of the class, the students and the healer give neck, shoulder and back massages to those attending.

During the class I asked for help with the bleeds. The points he called out were mostly familiar to me and made sense, especially L1-L3 and all five sacral nerves. The bleeds are decreasing in volume and have less blood in them now. Every so often, I muscle test to find out if I should be trying to stop them, and usually the answer has been no. One day, however, the answer was yes. I have a Chinese herb for this purpose, Yunnan Baiyao.

The problem at the bra line

I decided that I needed to give particular attention to the large osteophyte (bone spur) at T8-T9 that I had first seen on a full-spine X-ray taken in 1989, my first year in chiropractic school. How did I get it, and why should that be important? I have observed that, virtually without exception, women have a back problem at the bra line—around that level. I had also done a great deal of heavy lifting over the years in my former occupation as a stagehand. So the arthritis at that level had at least two biomechanical causes. T9 has been traditionally referred to as "stomach place" in chiropractic lore. I had noticed that when the bleeds were bad I would have severe gas as well as cramps and low back pain. I had also noticed that the gas improved if I adjusted the lower ribs for hiatal hernia.

It also stood to reason that the osteophyte could be causing nerve interference at the T8-T9 level, and that that would influence everything that went on below there—notably the ongoing bleeds. It's rather difficult to adjust the thoracics on oneself from the back, so I decided to do it from the front instead, using the ribs to shift the spine, as well as working with the spinous processes up as far as I could reach. This also has the advantage of adjusting the diaphragm, improving breathing and digestion, and freeing any piece of the stomach that might have gotten stuck in the hiatus in the diaphragm through which the esophagus passes. Since I've been working with this on a daily basis, I observe that the bleeds are beginning to decrease in duration and frequency. Cramping is much less severe than before. I think the improvement in rib function is responsible for that.

Dr. Arvigo's Maya Abdominal Massage also takes into account the importance of the upper abdomen in influencing the functioning or non-functioning of the uterus. I have found out first-hand how important this is.

I also think it likely that the ongoing nerve interference from this osteophyte is a major reason why the bleeding has gone on for so long. I do find that self-adjusting the lower ribs is helping.

Exit Wilhelmina

Jean was scheduled to return to Dutchess County on a Wednesday, having been delayed by that severe fall on Mother's Day, necessitating a hip replacement and surgical repair of a severely damaged left wrist. But she arrived from Florida on Monday, two days early. We all agreed that Wilhelmina the cat had called her. Jean and Karen both said that Wilhelmina wanted to make sure I was taken care of before she left the earth plane. I arranged for Jean, Shirley, and Teresa to stop in to say their farewells on Tuesday; Karen, Vicki, Jean and I would hold a circle for her on Wednesday, when Vicki and I had agreed to discontinue the hydration. At that time Wilhelmina could barely stand without falling over, and I remembered that a previous cat, Mr.Moose, had only lasted two more days after the staggering began.

What happened wasn't exactly what we expected. After the prayer circle, on Wednesday evening, she ate voraciously and showed an increased interest in life, even attempting to chase a bird when I set her down on the lawn near the nettle patch. She went back to the house and climbed the stairs by herself. The staggers decreased, although they didn't go away altogether. Vicki and I decided to resume hydration, and for another week at least she retained serious interest in food and stood up every time I came into the room. We didn't know quite what to make of it.

By Friday of the following week, she was weaker again, and she could barely walk when I set her down in the grass for the last time, in stark contrast to the week before. It was getting very difficult to interest her in food. Although she clearly wanted something, we couldn't find anything specific that she would eat.

Jean was coming in to be adjusted that day, and Wilhelmina came into the room with her, quite clearly wanting something, meowing and looking straight at her. At first she seemed confused as to whether she was supposed to "work on" Jean with the laying on of paws.

"Your work is done," Jean said, and told Patricia that Wilhelmina needed to talk to her. Patricia said that she had communicated with Wilhelmina a few days before, from a distance, but Jean said that wasn't good enough; Wilhelmina needed to look her in the eye and hear from her directly that Patricia would continue to be there for me.

Wilhelmina's last item of business

That day Patricia opened the door to find Wilhelmina standing shakily but purposefully there, looking up at her with what she describes as "laser eyes." She was waiting to hear what she needed to hear, and Patricia spoke to her aloud, from the heart.

Wilhelmina's laser eyes burned into her, and Patricia says she will never forget the intensity of that gaze.

This seems to have been the last piece of business Wilhelmina needed to accomplish before dying. I held her for a couple of hours. When I put her down, she was quite clearly not on the earth plane, apparently going ahead to see what was on the other side. When I came downstairs Saturday morning, she was unresponsive and chilled, although still alive. I held her from time to time during the day. Vicki came by around midday, and agreed with me not to hydrate. Patricia came by in the afternoon so that I wouldn't be alone.

I remembered that neither Mr. Moose nor Doc had left the earth plane in my presence; instead they had waited until I went away. So Patricia and I left for an hour or so. When we returned, Vicki was there to tell us that Wilhelmina was gone.

In this instance, the function of the two healing circles and the communications between Jean, Wilhelmina, and Patricia did not have the result of postponing death, but rather of allowing Wilhelmina to complete everything she needed to do, and to be reassured before dying. I am convinced that without the healing prayer and last visits from her friends, she would not have been able to go in peace. When Jean first returned from Florida, Wilhelmina, who Karen and I agreed was very close to dying, wasn't quite strong enough to complete things. The circles gave her the boost of energy she needed to orchestrate it perfectly.

This seems to be where this book should end. Old life ends, signaling a major shift, creating space for new life. The story, however, goes on. I continue learning and trying new things. I intend to work with Dr. Ulan's nutritional system on myself and some regular patients, comparing results with those from the Blood Test Evaluation and with information from the Standard

Process Symptom Survey. The Maya Abdominal Massage work is of tremendous importance to women, and I have found it to be a missing piece not adequately understood, either in chiropractic or in allopathic medicine. I continue to explore herbs and hope eventually to be able to use them instead of supplements in more situations, as I come to understand them better.

According to my muscle testing results, the cancer has been gone for four years now, but that does not mean that I can return to whatever bad habits I had before, or even that I would want to. I will continue to track it with the AMAS and may do one more ultrasound when the bleeding has stopped.

The reason for developing the cancer in the first place was to point out rather forcefully my need for change. I do not expect that it will recur, or that I will get another one, unless I slip into too many bad habits again. If this should happen, I know what to do.

I eagerly await reports from those of you who are working to heal yourselves of cancer without surgery, chemotherapy, radiation, or toxic and invasive diagnostic testing. The more of you, men and women, who take this approach to studying your own cancers and designing a treatment protocol based on enhancing health, the easier it will become for others to follow in your path. Designing cancer treatments to enhance life rather than focus on killing will become the norm, and will no longer be considered an aberration.

You are not alone.

PART III

Help Is at Hand

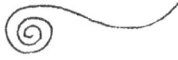

Thirty-four

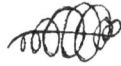

Toward an Individualized
Treatment of Cancer

*The Principles I Followed, Fourteen Possible Factors in
the Development of Cancer, and Some Trusted Protocols*

O nce you have been diagnosed with cancer, your life will
never be the same again—at least, hopefully not. If you
remain the same it will mean you haven't learned anything.

First, a word about—and perhaps a new view of—cancer.
Most people who are diagnosed with cancer have been conditioned to expect that it will inevitably kill them, and therefore are
frightened to death. This can become a self-fulfilling prophecy.
They tend to think that cancer comes out of nowhere, that it
strikes, is wild and uncontrollable, and doesn't relate in any way
to the behavior they have learned to expect from their bodies. I
am offering the good news that it is possible to reverse cancer
naturally; a cancer diagnosis is not necessarily a death sentence,
despite the prevailing attitudes in current Western culture.

As I mentioned before, cancer follows natural laws. Little
cancers are being formed by some sort of genetic error and

hunted down by the immune system all the time and will not generally get out of control if the individual is in good health. If they do get out of control, there are a number of potential reasons for this.

Also contrary to conventional thought, it is not always necessary to kill the cancer in order to heal from it. If, instead, you work conscientiously to improve your health, the cancer may well take care of itself.

The purpose of this chapter is to enumerate the possible causes of cancer and talk about ways in which they can be addressed.

A return to the beginning

I'm repeating myself a bit here, but it's important.

Cancer, described by the Chinese as "toxic heat with phlegm," is a distress call from the body, as I mentioned before. Physically, it is a progressive dedifferentiation of cells, a return to the beginning, the embryonic state, and is a default response to an intolerable situation, which could be physical or emotional. If you do not heed the call to change, the body will return to zero—in other words, it will die—*but it is perfectly willing to choose a different response if you're willing to work and negotiate with it.* Once the core problems have been recognized and are being dealt with, the illness has served its purpose. That doesn't mean you don't still have a lot of work to do.

The role of fear

Dr. Benhue He of China said, *"Fear of cancer is what kills."* Fear can cause you to make poor decisions precipitously. Most of the time, a week, two weeks, a month are usually not going to mean the difference between life and death—unless you *think* they are going to. Only occasionally is there an exception. Fear also sends hormonal messages to the body that can worsen your condition. It also may keep you from making a dispassionate analysis of your situation and responding rationally. Don't let anyone pressure you into a course of action that doesn't feel right.

Your response is one thing you can control

There are many circumstances that led up to your cancer. Some of these are more under your control than others. What you can always control is your response. Try to remember the Serenity Prayer, and have the courage to change the things you can. You may be surprised at how many things you can change. You don't have to change all of them at once. If you did, you wouldn't have any time left to live your life, and isn't that the point?

The more you are working the Fourteen Factors I will list here, the less you will need to rely on allopathic medicine's concepts of what your illness is and what you must do when. You will be more empowered.

It makes common sense that therapies should be pleasant and sustainable. After all, at the outset it is impossible to know for how long you may have to do them; it may be for a lifetime.

Some questions to consider

Some of the questions you need to consider when choosing treatments and therapies are these: Where has the cancer manifested? Is it progressing rapidly or slowly? Is it in a location where it threatens any aspect of breathing, eating, digestion, or circulation within the near future? What type is it? Has it metastasized or not? Is it in a location that offers a natural means of eliminating it?

The answers to these questions will indicate how much time is available to solve the problem. If time is short, it will be necessary to initiate more drastic therapies than if it is not. Nutritional building and detoxification are major elements of all natural therapies, but the proportion of nutritional building to detoxification and the intensity of the treatment vary widely.

FOURTEEN POSSIBLE FACTORS
IN THE DEVELOPMENT OF CANCER

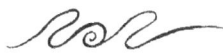

An individualized treatment of cancer begins, not with the cancer, but with consideration of the person who has it. S/he comes to it with a unique physical constitution, belief system, and set of experiences and current circumstances. Any treatment plan has to take these into account.

A good place to start plotting your own course is by asking, "Why me?" and answering this question honestly in terms of:

1. Your nutrition
2. The presence of toxicity, nutritional and environmental, in your life
3. Infection—bacterial, viral, parasitic, fungal
4. Your stress level
5. Your overall physical condition and genetic predisposition (which is *only* a predisposition)
6. Structural, biomechanical, ergonomic factors
7. Energetic factors
8. Sociologic cirumstances: presence/absence and quality of relationships with spouse/significant other, friends, family, business partners and co-workers; home
9. Your economic circumstances; work situation
10. Past unresolved emotional issues that may be triggered by current circumstances
11. Exercise and rest

12. Time you allow for pleasure, relaxation, spirituality, communion with nature
13. The amount of creative expression in your life
14. What do you think about the presence of cancer in your body? What does it mean to you?

When these fourteen "why me" questions have been answered, they will indicate the areas in need of change. How willing are you to make these changes? Each person has a unique balance of problems that will therefore require unique emphases in treatment. Cancer is generally a local manifestation of a systemic problem, and the "why me" questions should be answered in terms of both local and systemic issues.

Here, then, are expanded explanations of the fourteen things to take into account when choosing a treatment plan.

1) Nutrition

You are an individual unlike any other. So what is a perfect diet for someone else may not be right for you. Nutrition consists not only of diet, but also absorption, assimilation, elimination. The best diet in the world won't help if your body can't use it. Following are some strategies that will improve your general health and enhance digestion:

Nutritional therapies: juicing (especially carrot/apple), macrobiotics (for some people), supplementation, herbs, and dietary modification. In general, increase fruits and vegetables, reduce or eliminate sweets, fried foods, and anything not too easily digestible. Eat whole foods, locally grown, organic when possible, raw foods if your system can tolerate them. Cut out refined sugar, white flour, and other refined foods.

With regard to foods, the whole is more than the sum of its parts. Only in whole foods is there a natural synergy between the ingredients. Digestive enzymes will probably help, and are a part of many natural anti-cancer protocols. Probiotics help your digestive system do its work and reduce the number of unwanted proteins that cross from the gut into the bloodstream, thereby reducing the possibility of allergies and the load on your immune system. The Lactobacillus and other bacteria contained in yogurt are a common example; eating yogurt is one of the simplest and cheapest ways to create good digestion. Increase hydration, which is not only an issue of water intake but also of electrolyte balance. Proper hydration is essential for the movement of nutrients into and waste products out of the cell, for nerve function, for joint lubrication, for digestion.

As far as electrolytes go, ions with a positive charge are sodium and potassium; negatively-charged ones are chloride and bicarbonate. There should be a balance of both. Chloride goes to make hydrochloric acid, so if you run low on chloride, your stomach acid will be low. If your doctor gives you an antacid to relieve the gas this causes, it will make the problem worse. Slippery elm bark and rhubarb root, which are ingredients in the Essiac formula, are digestive aids. Eliminate foods to which you are allergic or sensitive. Listen to your body for specifics. Cancer loves sugar, as it works with anaerobic (not requiring oxygen) rather than aerobic metabolism. Cancer also has an affinity for iron, and it is preferable to get your iron from red meat or other food sources, rather than supplements, as much as you can.

Dr. Max Gerson stated that cancer begins with the liver and the digestion. (1). I think he was right. Therefore I question the long-term efficacy of any therapy that doesn't take this into account.

There is no one diet that is ideal for everyone. Dr. Peter D'Adamo discusses the different diets for the four blood types in *Eat Right for Your Type*. (2) I don't agree with all the specifics, and there are probably other moderating factors, but the concept makes sense to me. I have certainly encountered enough O blood type people who simply can't be vegetarians, so there must be something to it. However, it doesn't explain everything.

The conventional wisdom is that a vegetarian diet is good if you have cancer. My own experience tells me that this isn't always so. Look at any dietary imbalance you had prior to being diagnosed with the cancer, and correct it; if you were too far toward the carnivorous end of the spectrum, a vegetarian diet may be helpful, but if you have been too far toward the vegetarian end, you may have developed deficiencies that you need to correct, especially if you are an O blood type, are hypothyroid, or have been bleeding a lot as a result of your condition.

Your individuality will be reflected in your bloodwork, which can give indications of your nutritional issues. I used the Blood Test Evaluation by Health Equations, a computerized analysis of standard bloodwork that is then fine-tuned by your clinician's consultation with Lynne August, MD. If I were beginning the whole process now, I would begin with this or some other type of nutritional evaluation. It might be the most important thing you do.

2) Toxicity, nutritional and environmental

Toxicity in the air, in water, in soil, in food is becoming an increasingly severe problem, contributing to cancer and other degenerative diseases. Those with environmental illness and chemical sensitivities will need to pay particular attention to liver and bowel support. Recreational and medical drugs have to be cleared by the liver and/or kidneys, putting additional strain on these organs. Often these drugs work by inhibiting some natural process, and they may also deplete some necessary vitamins and minerals.

Alcohol puts additional stress on the liver, especially if you have a sensitivity to it. Other foods to which you are sensitive will also be stressful. If you smoke, quit. If you do caffeine, either cut down or quit. Once you begin detoxification, your metabolism will begin shifting. You may no longer be able to tolerate some of your old unhealthy habits.

Certain products applied to the skin (also hair dyes) may be a source of toxicity, especially underarm deodorants containing aluminum. The armpit has many lymph nodes close to the surface. Since the skin is a semipermeable membrane, the deodorant will be absorbed and taken up by the lymph nodes. Antiperspirants may thwart the body's attempt to get rid of toxins through perspiration. More research needs to be done on this as a possible contributing cause of breast cancer.

Some type of detoxification will probably be necessary. However, the worse your toxin load, the more gentle you have to be, the more slowly you have to work, and the more you have to build yourself up before attempting any kind of detoxification.

Detoxification methods include castor oil packs, liver-cleansing herbs, raw foods, colonics/enemas, chelation, fasting (sometimes). You may choose to have amalgam removed by a dentist who believes in and is conversant with biological dentistry; whether or not this is advisable varies with your individual situation, and it may not be an absolute prerequisite for healing. The amount of damage the mercury is doing to your system may be modulated by the acidity in your mouth. You may also choose to do it gradually to reduce the strain on your body and your finances. I have experienced an immediate increase in energy sometimes when an amalgam filling is removed, particularly if it was broken or leaking.

One of my correspondents, the daughter of a dental hygienist, tells me from personal experience that damage from mercury amalgam can be passed down as far as the third generation and can take many forms, including, but not limited to, brain tumors and other neurological and emotional problems.

Be aware of what toxic chemicals you may be using at home or work and see if you can come up with a more natural alternative. If not, increase protection.

3) Infection—bacterial, viral, parasitic, fungal

One or more infections may coexist with, or be a causative factor of, the cancer. Taking care of these reduces the burden on the body, making it easier for you to focus on healing. I found Dr. Hulda Clark's (3) parasite protocol helpful, despite never having been diagnosed with any parasites. It is inexpensive and low-risk.

If you are using antibiotics, you will then have to deal with a fungal overgrowth, because antibiotics will kill off both useful and pathogenic bacteria, allowing the fungus to grow unimpeded. So be sure to use probiotics during any course of antibiotics.

Bacterial or viral infections can cause inflammation in the gut, thereby increasing its permeability. This means that toxins or undigested proteins can get into the blood more easily, and your immune system will mount a defense. This may cause allergic reactions. Acidophilus has a normalizing effect on the gut. It produces B complex and helps your gut deal with food poisoning and reduces the burden on the immune system.

I found castor oil packs very helpful in taking care of fungal infections.

4) Stress level

Your body responds to stress by producing cortisol. Cortisol reduces your immune response, because it is designed to clear up the debris from the inflammatory process. This is intended as a short-term response only. Long-term stress and consequent overproduction of cortisol can lead to osteoporosis, among other things.

Design your therapy according to your specific stressors. Most people I have talked to who developed cancer had some major life stressor(s) in the two or three years prior to diagnosis. In some cases, an injury caused nerve interference to the area. (If so, address this structurally, using chiropractic or other mechanical therapies, and energetically, using acupuncture, Reiki, or some other form of energy work.) Address the problems as directly as possible. Use talk therapy. In addition to altered hormonal levels related to stress, self-care has a tendency to go out the window. Reestablish whatever self-care routines you had formerly that you have discontinued. Practice meditation, exercise, especially yoga and/or Tai Chi/qigong, things you like to do. Stop watching the news and violent shows on television. Not only does there tend to be a lot of negativity on TV, but watching the screen itself can be overstimulating and create a sleep disturbance. This can also be true of computer use. I find pinhole glasses helpful to minimize the glare of the screen.

If you are currently using caffeine, nicotine, or alcohol, these are also raising your stress level. Now might be a good time to stop.

5) Overall physical condition and genetic predisposition (which is only a predisposition)

By definition, if you've been diagnosed with cancer, you're not in tiptop shape, but you could be anywhere along the continuum. There is always room for improvement, so work on improving your general health, especially nutrition, hydration, exercise, rest. If you have a genetic predisposition, try not to repeat your ancestors' mistakes.

6) Structural, biomechanical, ergonomic factors

The health of the spine influences the input of the nervous system into the organs; they can overfunction or underfunction as a result. The longer the nerves have been irritated, the more potentially dangerous the situation is. Poor blood and lymph circulation can result in the hypoxia (too little oxygen) of muscles and organs and poor waste removal, which can cause toxicity. Muscle tension cuts down on the blood supply. Cancer thrives in an anaerobic (low or no oxygen) environment, whereas normal cells do not. In other words, as I have said earlier, cancer can arise from a situation of cell starvation.

Adjusting the spine and massaging the muscles increase oxygenation and perfusion (blood feeding the structure) as well as improve nerve function. I may tend to underplay the importance of this because, as a chiropractor, I sometimes take it for granted. A friend of mine developed cervical cancer some time after an injury that caused a lumbar disc herniation. "Do you think they were related?" I asked. "You bet," she said. The lumbar disc problem created chronic muscle spasm, pain and numbness down the leg to the foot, a result of nerve interference. Sexual organs are innervated (receive nerve impulses) from the sacrum, below the level of the disc herniation. She also briefly lost bowel control shortly after the injury.

Analyze ergonomics and see if your clothing is binding. Bras may be a contributing factor in breast cancer, because they can impede the flow of lymph.

Motion of the ribs tends to become more restricted as people grow older, due to chronic spasm of the intercostals (muscles between the ribs), thereby decreasing the capacity of the lungs and restricting motion of the heart. Holding the breath is a common response to pain. The older one is, the more old injuries one is likely to have, and the more likely one is to be subconsciously restricting breathing as protection against old pain. Adjusting the ribs can release old physical and emotional pain patterns.

Yoga and qigong are powerful tools for increasing oxygen to the tissues, because of their emphasis on the breath. This is tremendously important, because cancer arises in a state of low oxygen, but the importance of the breath tends to be neglected in Western cultures.

7) Energetic factors

Energy is a difficult area to define specifically—an area where body and spirit overlap. Are you allowing people and situations to drain your energy? Acupuncture, qigong, Reiki, yoga and other active and passive energetic therapies realign the way your energy flows and the way you respond to the world. Feng shui is important because the energetic state of your surroundings reflects the energetic state of your body.

8) Sociologic circumstances: presence/absence and quality of relationships with spouse/significant other, friends, family, business partners and co-workers; home

Who is your community? Analyze its strengths and weaknesses. It may have a lot to offer you in terms of tangible help as well as emotional support.

Is your relationship supporting or draining you?

Are you living where you want to? Or are you there out of a sense of obligation to someone else? Is the place you live supporting or draining you?

Talk therapy and twelve-step groups are opportunities to examine these areas and work on whatever you perceive to be lacking. You're going to need your support system, so clue them in on your situation. Conversely, don't waste your energy trying to convince those who don't agree with the way you've chosen to treat your condition; you need energy to heal. Prayer and healing circles are excellent. Three important factors in making prayer effective are intention, visualization, and expectation. You must expect that it will work. Praying in the name of your Higher Power, whoever it may be, gives direction and force to your prayer, and thanking your Higher Power for working on your problem creates in you the expectation that your prayer will be answered. Adding the intention, visualization and expectation of others to your own increases the power of your prayer. The answer may not be given precisely as you thought it would, so don't try to give your Higher Power too much direction.

The answers to your prayer may be other people. Don't be afraid to ask; people are more than willing to give help and advice. There are many out there who have already succeeded at what you are trying to do.

Are you happy? If not, why not? You are responsible for your own happiness. Do your own research; draw your own conclusions. Take control of your situation and your life.

9) Economic circumstances, work situation

Self-explanatory. This is a HUGE factor! Economic limitations are one of the biggest stress factors contributing to cancer. It is undeniably easier to heal your cancer if you have economic resources, but that doesn't mean it's impossible if you don't.

You still have a wide variety of simple and inexpensive therapies open to you. If you have a yard not being treated with chemicals, it probably contains a number of edible and medicinal herbs that won't cost you a dime. Learn about these and incorporate them into your regime.

Call for help; don't be a hero. Your life is more important than your paycheck. If you don't have health, you can't work, so take care of health first and the economics will catch up when you're feeling better. There is a danger point when the initial crisis is past and you are resuming the duties and complexities of everyday life. Don't rush this process.

There's probably something in this area that needs to change, and you probably know what it is. If you hate your job, quit or change it. If your stomach clenches every day when you go in to work, this is a biological imperative that you ignore at your peril. If economics make it impossible at this time, don't despair, but you must at least begin to plot your way out.

10) Past unresolved emotional issues that may be triggered by current circumstances

Again, try talk therapy. Also, any form of therapy that accesses an altered state will help you cut through a lot of garbage much faster than straight talk therapy, especially if you've gone over the same ground before. Guided Imagery and Music, EMDR (Eye Movement Desensitization and Reprocessing), and hypnosis are some of these. The Enneagram may be useful, as are healing prayer and healing circles. The specific form doesn't matter, so long as it helps you get at what's been bothering you—there has to be something! You want to access your higher self and Divine Intelligence, so divination in whatever form you like is terrific, so long as you don't become dependent on it. Learn as much as you can. Take control of your situation. Don't panic. Your thoughts will shape the course of your healing, so be mindful of them and change those that are self-defeating. Edgar Cayce said, "Spirit is the life, mind is the builder, the physical is the result."

Bodywork and energy therapies such as Reiki are important here. The body has a story to tell. You may not be able to access this by talk alone.

Your dreams may contain important information about your healing or give you an indication of what problems you need to solve. Pay attention to them. Write them down as soon as you can, before you wake up totally and they vanish.

Dr. Bernie Siegel in *Love, Medicine and Miracles* and *Peace, Love and Healing* describes the use of drawings to elicit the body's assessment of the illness and unconscious attitudes toward the planned therapy (4).

Face your own mortality. This is a major lesson of this condition. I find the Tibetans especially helpful, particularly *The Tibetan Book of Living and Dying* by Sogyal Rinpoche(5).Once you've addressed this issue, there's a lot less to be afraid of.

Accept where you are at the moment. It is the starting point of your journey. Once you become accepting, rather than struggling, it is easier to discern what needs to change and to change it.

11) Exercise and rest

Do what the body tells you. Probably you haven't been getting enough rest, and this may well have been an important factor in creating your condition. Rest is not only sleep; it is also whatever replenishes you.

Life is motion. The body is designed to have bursts of intense physical activity alternating with periods of rest. It would appear that this is a simple principle, but in fact Western culture seems to be attempting to edit both exercise and rest out of life and substitute—what? Sustained mental activity and stimulation combined with physical slothfulness, with no time to rest and reset. This is dangerous and probably has had a hand in causing your illness and those of many of your friends or family. Human beings aren't designed to function this way, so many rely on energy drinks or other stimulants to keep going at a faster pace than they're designed for and pain killers to allow them to ignore the body's signals to stop.

Overstimulation results in sleep deprivation. This in turn leads to errors in cell division and impairs the responsiveness of your immune system.

I find it necessary to avoid computers or television (electronic stimulation) late at night. Sleep disturbances can also result from hypoglycemia or mineral deficiency. Ayurvedic herbalists recommend adding ashwagandha to the old standby warm milk and honey at bedtime. (I often use yogurt and maple syrup in order to obtain the added benefits of *Lactobacillus.*) You should also take your calcium and magnesium in the evening, as minerals are sedative. Avoid caffeine in the evening. Don't go to bed angry.

12) Time allowed for pleasure, relaxation, spirituality, communion with nature

Stress makes one neglectful of these areas. The more you're enjoying your life, the more you'll be inclined to go on living it.

Alienation from nature is arguably the single greatest cause of disease. We were designed to live in nature, in cooperation with other forms of life, but we seem to have forgotten this, preferring to use technology to distance ourselves from each other and from our plant and animal neighbors. Your individual illness may be a symptom of this collective one.

As mentioned before, healing prayer is important, not only as emotional support, but it often works, especially when intention, visualization and expectation are strong—sometimes dramatically and immediately, often more subtly and over time, and not necessarily exactly as you originally envisioned. I find that it helps get my consciousness out of the way and let the body and Universal Intelligence do what they do best.

13) Creative expression

What is the mark you intend to leave on the world? Stop putting it off. Act on it. Take more emotional risks than usual. Hopefully your condition is serving to light a fire under you.

14) What do you think about the presence of cancer in your body? What does it mean to you?

It has been established that your attitude *can* alter your biology.

SOME ESTABLISHED,
TRUSTED NATURAL PROTOCOLS

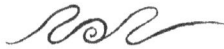

A protocol is a collection of therapies. After you have considered the fourteen questions, you have several choices as to what you are going to do with your cancer. You can:

1. Heal or eliminate it
2. Wall it off
3. Let it stay more or less as it is for a greater or lesser period of time; speed it up or slow it down
4. Let it get away on you, metastasize and possibly kill you
5. Reverse it to a greater or lesser extent

Once you have decided on one of these goals, there are many strategies available to you for implementing it.

The degree of nutritional building, detoxification and rest needed, for instance, is highly variable and can be determined by careful evaluation of the "why me" answers with a health care professional who has a strong grounding in nutrition. (Even if you yourself are a health care professional with a strong grounding in nutrition, you need someone else to check your work and think of things you've missed.) Your overall condition will be improved by nutritional building, detoxification and rest. *Your goal is to make yourself too healthy to be sick.* If your condition has consequences, such as chronic bleeding, take steps to replace the nutrients lost.

Therapies involving nutritional building are:

1. Careful evaluation of diet, with particular attention to increasing fresh vegetables and fruits, the more colorful the better;
2. Use of tonifying herbs
3. Vitamin and mineral supplementation
4. Seaweeds, blue-green algae, spirulina, chlorella
5. Juicing.

Most of the best-known nutritional protocols include elements of, or are combinations of, the above. Some of these are

1) **Macrobiotics.** I don't have much personal experience with this but it appears to eliminate just about all allergens and irritants from the diet as well as being rich in greens and seaweeds, always a good thing. Calls for little to no animal protein. Cooking and food preparation are very important, so macrobiotics is not for someone who doesn't have time for or doesn't want to prepare and cook. May not be suitable for someone who requires meat.

2) **Essiac**, a combination of herbs (sheep sorrel, burdock root, slippery elm bark, and turkey rhubarb root) originally used by the Ojibway Indians and brought to public attention by Rene Caisse, a Canadian nurse. (6) A more recent formulation, FlorEssence, also includes potentiating herbs, watercress, blessed thistle, red clover, and kelp. There are many versions on the market, some better than others. I have been told that having the correct sheep sorrel (*Rumex acetosella*) is particularly important. I like this formula because it contains common herbs indigenous

to the area I live in. Besides, my experience is that it works, gently, to rebuild the body. I find that it improves glucose tolerance, an important issue with cancer. The taste is pleasant.

3) **The Hoxsey formula**, another herbal formula developed by Harry Hoxsey, originating from his grandfather's observation of the herbs chosen by a horse who had a cancer on his leg. There are about ten herbs in the Hoxsey formula, some of which are more toxic than those in Essiac and should therefore be used with more caution.

4) **Gerson** is a strict regime involving extensive use of juicing, coffee enemas and supplementation, based on the work of Max Gerson, MD and explained in detail in his book, *A Cancer Therapy: Results of Fifty Cases.* (7) Gerson has been effective in curing metastasized melanoma, something conventional medicine says can't be done. This is quite an intense therapy and requires a total commitment, and if you're very sick, you'll need help. Dr. Gerson's daughter, Charlotte, wrote a less technical description, *The Gerson Therapy: The Amazing Nutritional Program for Cancer and Other Illnesses* (8). Further information is available from the Gerson Institute. (see Resources)

5) **Kelley** (has similarities to Gerson) Emphasizes the use of enzymes to aid in protein metabolism, which he believed was deficient in cancer patients, Postulated a relationship between trypsin (an enzyme factor in digestion) and malignin, which is an indicator of the presence of cancer. Had a four-point program including coping with issues of spirit. (9)

6) **Dr. Emanuel Revici** postulated the **lipid defense** as an oscillation between catabolic and anabolic processes, inflammatory (fatty acids) and anti-inflammatory (sterols) compounds. He discerned two distinct pain patterns, alkaline and acid pain, and sought to use these to tailor therapies to the individual. (10)

Therapies involving detoxification are:

- Liver: castor oil packs, adequate hydration, herbs, yoga, qigong, protein, rest
- Bowel: castor oil packs, adequate hydration, probiotics, enemas/colonics, high fiber diet, yoga, qigong; parasite cleanse, as described by Hulda Clark, N.D. in *The Cure for All Cancers* (11)
- Kidney: adequate hydration, herbs, electrolytes
- Lungs: exercise, especially yoga or qigong, which emphasize the breath; deep breathing. Chiropractic or osteopathic adjustment to mobilize the ribs
- Skin: brushing and cleansing the skin, exercise, sauna, sweat lodge, steam bath, or whirlpool
- Systemic: Removal of dental amalgam; chelation.

Many nutritional therapies also detoxify.

This list is by no means exhaustive. There is a wide spectrum of alternative cancer therapies. It would be impossible to do all of them in a lifetime, even if you did nothing else, so don't even try. The number and variety of approaches can be bewildering at first. My general rule is, if a therapy doesn't appeal to you, don't use it—the body is telling you it isn't the right one at this time.

A popular misconception is that all alternative therapies are expensive. Nothing could be further from the truth. Some of the best ones are either cheap or free. There is nothing to stop you from selecting the elements of a specific program that you like, skipping the rest of it, and substituting other things to accomplish the same goals less expensively.

Useful books and periodicals

The best overview I found is *Cancer Diagnosis: What to Do Next*, by Drs. Diamond and Cowden and Burton Goldberg (12). Jean's Greens in Castleton Corners, New York, offers a *Review of Herbal Cancer Therapies* by C.J. Puotinen, which is excellent. (13)

Herbalist and nutritionist Donald R. Yance, Jr. has worked with cancer for many years and has written *Herbal Medicine, Healing and Cancer*, (14) also available from Jean's Greens. *The Townsend Letter* usually has an issue devoted to cancer twice a year and a regular column on *The War on Cancer* by Ralph Moss in every issue. (15) You will find some very provocative articles on subjects studiously avoided in the mainstream press and a lot of very fine scientific writing.

About diagnostic testing

Find out from your doctor—and research on your own—the potential toxicity of any diagnostic tests you are contemplating. Do they involve either radiation or injected radioactive contrast media, or both? This is particularly germane if you have already been treated with radiation. (Some patients have described to me their progressively worsening reactions to CT scans in particular. My feeling is, the fewer of these, the better. I personally will not use them, at all.) If so, can you do a less invasive test and find out close to the same thing? Or, do you really need a test right now?

About staging

If your cancer was discovered through a routine screening test, you may need further testing to learn more about it. How much do you need to know? Your doctor, especially if s/he is an oncologist, may advise you to have the cancer staged. Staging is a method of describing the location and spread (or not) of the cancer, according to a system using Roman numerals and letters. The meaning varies according to the type of cancer described, but generally, the higher a number the Roman numeral is, the more widespread the cancer is.

If you are having surgery to remove the organ in question, it is quite likely that the cancer will be staged, because then the pathologist has a nice tissue sample to work with, which will automatically be analyzed during the course of the surgery. If you are NOT having surgery, however, staging will require expensive and invasive diagnostic testing such as CT scans. Ultrasound is not precise enough to accomplish this.

Do you really need the information about location and spread that this will give you, or will the use of radiation and radioactive contrast media—and the expense— cause more trouble than it's worth? Will the result, whatever it is, change your course of action? If you have some handle on how you're feeling and have been using the AMAS and ultrasounds, you may not need additional information. Staging is most useful if you are debating surgery. Otherwise, how much you need to know is a highly individual decision.

About mammography

I question the use of mammography as a screening test. A good screening test should be noninvasive and cheap; mammography is neither. In my opinion, the danger of radiation increases with repetition. Recent research bears this out. Rose Marie Williams addresses this issue in the August/September 2007 *Townsend Letter (*16). According to Ms. Williams, "The increased cancer risk from mammography was well-established before the NCI and the American Cancer Society (ACS) launched their large-scale screening of pre-menopausal women in the 1970s." (17) Yet the ACS is still recommending annual screening. Why? Radiation can induce a cancer as well as detect one. There is also the question of false positives leading to unnecessary biopsies. Thermography and ultrasound have potential as safer options. Mammography may still have value in determining the nature of a lesion discovered by other means. Nutritionist John Cartmell comments, "Having an annual mammogram is like jumping on the roof checking for leaks. Eventually you'll find one." (18)

Testing for the presence of cancer with the AMAS

The AMAS (anti-malignin antibody in serum, done by Oncolab in Boston) is a blood test that appears to indicate the presence of cancer of any type. The antibody titer is elevated in the presence of active cancer and returns to normal if the cancer is treated successfully or if it is terminal and the body can no longer mount an immune response. This test can be especially useful in place of or in corroboration of a more invasive test, especially if the possible cancer site is inaccessible. The antibody level seems to drop sharply between day 90 and day 97 post-surgery. (19) My experience has told me, however, that it may take as long as four months for the antibody titer to drop after surgery.

Oncolab will mail you a free information packet and a free test kit, if you ask for them.

I live in New York State. New York State has more stringent regulations governing laboratories than other states, and out-of-state labs may not wish to comply with them. One time I was told that Oncolab could not mail test kits to an address in New York State, but this has not been a problem recently. I had my blood draw done in Connecticut. Be sure to tell your phlebotomist not to use a butterfly to do the draw, because the plastic tubing will lower the antibody titer by 10-30 points. Oncolab states this in their instructions to the lab (on the sheet of paper with your name and information and your doctor's), but there is no guarantee that your phlebotomist has read them. The test requires about three hours of handling by the lab where the draw is done, and then needs to be shipped in dry ice to Oncolab the same day. You may need to call the lab in advance to order the dry ice. The draw needs to be done Monday through Thursday, so that the sample can arrive at Oncolab the next day, since freezing overnight adversely affects the accuracy of the test. Go to the blood draw site in the early morning to make sure they have plenty of time to process the sample before the daily FedEx shipment goes out. Bring a FedEx slip with you and a credit card number; you have to pay the shipping.

Linda Strega comments that there have been problems getting samples to Oncolab from the West Coast without their thawing en route. If you're on the West Coast, talk to your lab about this before having your doctor order the test. Oncolab now has information on labs in your area that can perform the draw and doctors who use this test, if you call the Oncolab central number. From my experience, not many mainstream MDs are familiar with this invaluable test.

If you're still not sure what to do...

If the AMAS titer is elevated, and you are not in acute distress, take some measures to improve general health and repeat the test in about three months. I find the usefulness of this test increases with repetition. If you still haven't brought the titer down to normal, and you're not quite sure where the problem is, it might be helpful to seek out a medical intuitive to narrow your search and help you focus on what your body is trying to tell you. Edgar Cayce was the earliest and best-documented medical intuitive of recent times. Norman Shealy, MD collaborated with Caroline Myss on research into medical intuition. Medical intuitives are becoming more common and respected, and the quality of medical intuition is improving. Ask people you know and trust to get a referral. The use of medical intuition may help you avoid a panel of toxic, invasive and expensive diagnostic tests. If you're in serious trouble, a medical intuitive may help you figure out your next steps.

Types of interventions; how your body is tuned

Hopefully you have had sufficient experience with healing other conditions to know what type of interventions work best for you. From the most subtle to the most aggressive, these are:

1. Nutrition, which is a given.
2. Homeopathy, vibrational remedies, flower essences, energy work, sound
3. Herbs, qigong, yoga, other forms of exercise

4. Supplements, massage, chiropractic, acupuncture
5. Drugs
6. Surgery, radiation, chemotherapy

If your body is tuned to subtler modalities, drugs, surgery, chemo and radiation may be too violent for you. If you have been accustomed to drugs and surgery, on the other hand, subtler modalities may not work.

In my readings on the subject, I have observed two patterns. One is that most nonallopathic interventions that are said to "fight cancer" seem to work on the principle of building the immune system or aiding digestion. But some herbal remedies do act on the principle of "killing" errant cells. Herbal or not, they are cytotoxic. The Taxol family of chemotherapy drugs, for example, is derived from the Pacific yew, a plant. However, if you are using herbs with the goal of killing cancer in mind, you are simply duplicating the Western medical wartime mindset, with its attendant liabilities.

Recovery from conventional cancer treatments: drawbacks

The other pattern I've found is that a discussion of nutritional recovery from cancer that has been treated by conventional means will generally focus on recovery from the *treatment* and not from the cancer. It surprises me that more authors do not question or comment on the phenomenon of limiting the healing power of nutrition in this way. When I went to bookstores looking for information on using nutrition to treat cancer, all I found were books on nutritional recovery, not from cancer, but from conventional treatments. It's beginning to dawn on the general public, however, that allopathic "treatments" are killing patients faster than cancer.

To compensate for the anemia resulting from chemo or radiation, your doctor might prescribe an epoetin—a drug intended to boost kidney production of the hormone that induces the production of red blood cells—though now it appears that these also may be highly unsafe as well as expensive. (20) Try to find the recovery in this pattern: cancer treated with toxicity produces anemia, which is treated with more toxicity, leading to the possibility of stroke. One author, Donald Yance, Jr. outlines herbal and nutritional support for both cancer and treatment recovery in *Herbal Medicine, Healing and Cancer* (21).

The wartime mentality: drawbacks

There is no reason why the rules for healing cancer should be any different than the rules for healing any other condition. Because there are so many factors, physical and otherwise, leading up to cancer, it is unlikely that anyone will ever find a single "magic bullet." So why does everyone keep looking for "the cure"? Upon analysis of the "why me?" questions, it becomes clear that cancer, unlike Lyme disease, comes from self and not from outside and can arise from a multiplicity of causes. It is one's own cells that have gone awry. So "war on cancer" is war on self. You may remember that Dr. Gladys McGarey, in talking about Living Medicine, describes how modern allopathic medicine was shaped during World War II. (22) Therefore the language of conventional medicine is full of such words as "kill," "battle," and "destroy." War, as everyone knows, is a costly and exhausting process, and it is questionable whether anyone ever really wins it. I think it preferable not to wage war at all, but instead to get to know and understand your cancer in all of its complexities.

I suspect that, even if the theories of causation by a bacterium/virus (Rife) or intestinal parasites (Hulda Clark) are ultimately proven to be correct, it will also be found that these organisms are ubiquitous and cosmopolitan—all over the place inside us, whether or not there is any active disease— and that susceptibility to disease will still be a matter of host susceptibility or resistance due to the above factors. I also suspect that different organisms can promote different cancers in different hosts at different times, that there is not necessarily a single universal cause.

Royal Rife designed a series of microscopes that made it possible for him to look at live specimens under the lens with far higher resolutions and magnifications than had ever been achieved before. He used light to stain them rather than the stains commonly used, which will kill the specimens being observed. In the course of his investigations, he discovered that the same organism could at one time be a rod-shaped bacterium, at another time, a round bacterium, and at another time could be a filterable virus (pleomorphism) thereby setting conventional microbiology on its ear.

Rife had trouble with the medical establishment, a pattern I have observed repeatedly, and therefore pleomorphism is still not commonly taught. He discovered through repeated observation that bacteria could be destroyed—exploded—by subjecting them to electrical frequencies specific to the organism. Using these principles, he successfully treated cancer in an experimental clinic in 1934. (23) The "Rife Machine," a device that generates the frequencies to destroy bacteria, is now being used experimentally in the treatment of Lyme disease.

What should your doctor do for you?

You hire your doctor to do a job for you, which includes analyzing your situation, giving advice, listening to you, honoring your choices and/or suggesting what might work better, authorizing whatever you might need in the way of diagnostic testing to follow your protocol and treating you if you are in agreement with the style of treatment s/he offers. A doctor who is not conversant with holistic medicine not only may not counsel you on the above interventions, s/he may never have heard of them and may therefore discount them as useless. Be prepared to do your own research and be aware that you may know more about this topic than your doctor does.

If s/he does not do this job to your satisfaction, fire that one and hire another.

If, instead, you choose conventional treatment

If you have chosen one of the conventional therapies, it will cause serious nutritional depletion, among other things, for which you will have to compensate. Conventional treatments are designed to inhibit a pathological process, NOT to enhance health! Some types of chemotherapy are antimetabolites—they interfere with some natural process, hoping thereby to starve the cancer before they starve you. If you're doing chemo or radiation, work with a nutritionist who is familiar with these modalities to replace some of what you're losing. So-called "side effects" are the result of the interference with metabolism that is supposed to be "killing cancer" injuring healthy cells as well. There is a lot of controversy about using supplements during chemo or radiation.

Some studies point to Chinese herbs and some Western herbs as being useful with chemo and radiation. (24) If you're not sure, Dr. Jody Noe (25) recommends not supplementing for three days before and three days after the treatment as a general rule.

If you're choosing surgery, particularly for breast or uterine cancers, removal of lymph nodes is commonly done. Beware! Any doctor who removes a lot of lymph nodes that turn out to be healthy isn't doing you a favor. Your immune system will never work as well again; your circulation won't be right; you will have to deal with swelling of the affected extremity and be very careful of cuts, contact dermatitis, or any potential source of infection. Lymph nodes that are biopsied are gone forever, healthy or not. Discuss with your surgeon beforehand the usefulness of a "sentinel node" biopsy in your case. S/he will take a "sentinel node" and biopsy that, figuring that if it is healthy, the others surrounding it are healthy also. This usually works, but not 100% of the time. A dye may also be used to test lymph nodes.

Lymphatics are a major component of the immune defense and of the circulation, and destroying them can lead to development of more cancers later on, which the body will not be able to handle. Sometimes your doctor will suggest radiation instead, in order to avoid this problem, but radiation can also destroy lymphatic circulation and can also give rise to leukemia. It isn't even effective for some types of cancer, but may be recommended anyway. Recent studies indicate that radiation used for breast cancer may cause heart damage. (26) Radiation works by creating free radicals, which you spend the rest of your time trying to avoid.

After your surgery, you may wish to have an AMAS (antimalignin antibody in serum) blood test done to find out whether or not you are cancer free. As I noted before, it will take about 97 days after surgery for the antibody levels to fall, which they should do if your treatment was successful, according to Oncolab's literature. (27) Again, my experience is that it may take as long as four months for the antibody titer to drop. Oncolab recommends waiting for at least a month after the end of chemotherapy to test antibody levels.

Remission or cure?

To treat cancer nonallopathically, you need to have a high tolerance for ambiguity.

Probably the most difficult aspect is the lack of a definite end point, whereas if you've had surgery, radiation, or chemo, the theory is that you don't have any more cancer after that. Sometimes this works. Sometimes it doesn't. When does it work? Say that before your illness your health is at 8/10. Surgery without complications may bring it down to 5/10. Are you cancer-free? Maybe. Are you healthy? No. Then you have chemo or radiation, bringing it down to 3/10. Are you cancer-free? Maybe. Are you healthy? Definitely not! Remember that little cancers are starting up in your body all the time, and your immune system is supposed to be hunting them down and getting rid of them. Unfortunately, chemo or radiation has compromised your immune system. You may be in remission, but unless you get your health back up to 7/10, you cannot be "cured." (28)

The bottom line

When you're treating by natural means, sometimes you will feel better. Sometimes you will feel worse. Sometimes you'll know whether your condition is improving. Sometimes you won't. And every choice you make and every belief you have has the potential to alter its course.

So what's the bottom line?

- Eat real food. Make everything you eat count.
- Clean up your act.
- Rest.
- Exercise.
- Get light and air.
- Communicate with your Higher Power.
- Connect with, love and support your neighbors, human, plant and animal.

Doesn't this sound like what your mother told you?

Thanks to Linda Strega and John Cartmell, whose comments have been addressed in this revision.

REFERENCES FOR THIS CHAPTER

1. Gerson, Max, MD, *A Cancer Therapy: Results of Fifty Cases,* Del Mar, California: Totality Books, 1958, p.35

2. D'Adamo, Peter, ND, *Eat Right 4 Your Type*, New York: G.P. Putnam's Sons, 1996

3. Clark, Hulda Regehr, Ph.D, ND, *The Cure for All Cancers,* Chula Vista, CA: New Century Press, 1993

4. Siegel, Bernie, MD, *Love, Medicine & Miracles,* New York, NY: Harper & Row, 1986, 1990

5. --------------------, *Peace, Love & Healing,* NY: HarperCollins, 1989

6. Rinpoche, Sogyal, *The Tibetan Book of Living and Dying,* San Francisco, CA: Harper Collins, 2002

7. Thomas, Richard, *The Essiac Report,* Los Angeles, CA: The Alternative Treatment Information Network, 1993

8. Gerson, Max, *A Cancer Therapy*

9. Gerson, Charlotte, and Walker, Morton, DPM, *The Gerson Therapy: The Amazing Nutritional Program for Cancer and Other Illnesses,* New York, NY: Kensington Publishing, 2001

10. Roberts, Melina A., "A Critique of the Kelley Nutritional-Metabolic Cancer Program," *Townsend Letter,* June 2003, p.26

11. Revici, Emanuel, MD, *Research in Physiopathology as Basis of Guided Chemotherapy,* 1961. Available from Health Equations

12. Clark, Hulda Regehr, ND, *The Cure for All Cancers*

13. Diamond, John, MD, Cowden, Lee, MD, and Goldberg, Burton, *Cancer Diagnosis: What to Do Next,* Tiburon, CA: Alternative Medicine.com, 2000

14. Puotinen, CJ, *A Review of Herbal Cancer Therapies,* Schodack, NY: Jean's Greens, 2000

15. Yance, Donald R. and Valentine, Arlene, *Herbal Medicine, Healing and Cancer,* Lincolnwood, IL: Keats Publishing, 1999

16. *Townsend Letter,* Port Townsend, WA

17. Williams, Rose Marie, "X-Rays and Mammograms Increase Cancer Risk," *Townsend Letter,* August/September 2007, p.56-61

18. *Ibid,* p. 57

19. Cartmell, John, personal communication

20. Abrams, p.74

21. Moss, Ralph, Ph.D, "Oncologists Are Paid to Prescribe Dubious Drugs" *Townsend Letter,* August/September 2007, p.52-55

22. Yance and Valentine, *Herbal Medicine, Healing and Cancer*

23. Gladys McGarey, MD, speaking on the subject of Living Medicine, The Crossings, Austin, TX, May 2007

24. Lynes, Barry, *The Cancer Cure That Worked!* Queensville, Ontario, Canada: Marcus Books, 1987

25. Yance and Valentine, *Herbal Medicine, Healing and Cancer*

26. Noe, Jody, ND, *Herbs and Cancer,* International Herb Symposium, Norton, MA, June 2007

27. Moss, Ralph, Ph.D, "Big Blow to Radiation for Breast Cancer," *Townsend Letter,* Port Townsend, WA, July 2007, p.58-60

28. Abrams, Martin B. *et al.,* "Early Detection and Monitoring of Cancer with the Anti-Malignin Antibody Test," *Cancer Detection and Prevention*, 18-(1): 65-78, 1994

29. Cartmell, John, personal communication

When Is It Too Late?

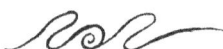

I've been asked to address the question: When is it too late? When does it become impossible to change an inevitable slide toward death?

I don't know the answer. It's beyond my experience. The more I become aware of the miraculous changeability of the body, the farther off this point seems.

Yet, as Bernie Siegel reminds us, life is terminal.

Sometimes the end is sudden, allowing for no discussion or debate. We can be taken out at any time.

The end occurs when the heart no longer beats, when breathing or brain activity stops. If a tumor obstructs breathing, makes eating impossible, or tears through an artery, causing hemorrhage, this can be an end-point. Technological advances have changed the end-point in many cases and have also allowed for the increased incidence of near-death experiences. Some people return not only with a glimpse of the other side, but also with new strength, power, and conviction—and, in the case of Mellen-Thomas Benedict, the disappearance of the condition that killed him for ninety minutes.

What's going on here?

Does metastasis to bone make the condition incompatible with life? Not necessarily, though the compromising of the bone marrow, where blood is made, makes this a particularly difficult situation. One necessary task, on the physical level, is to flood the body with nutrition to compensate for the decreased carrying capacity of the blood. When the richly innervated periosteum is disrupted by tumors, deep pain can result. This saps the energy and is severely demoralizing.

Remember, however, that cancer is a default response. What are the possibililties when the body's cries for change are finally heeded?

"Where there's life, there's hope."

I know of a couple of instances of people with remissions of cancer that ultimately didn't last. In both cases, they had remained in difficult relationships. Did the remissions not last because they had not listened to the body's cries for change?

Some who have reported near-death experiences say they were given a choice to remain on the other side or to return. Others were told that it wasn't their time yet.

I've observed people and cats choosing their time. I have seen several cats choose to leave the planet in late summer or early fall, knowing that winter is coming on and not wanting to endure another one. They seem to make their choice either by stopping eating or running in front of cars, probably one of the few methods of suicide available to them.

Many authors have remarked on the phenomenon that people often hang on until after major holidays and arrange to see everyone important in their lives as much as possible before making their transitions. My mother did that, making sure that everyone would be gathered for Thanksgiving.

I think the choice of how much pain is too much, or how much physical disintegration is too much, is as individual as the "bottom" in alcoholism or addiction. For one alcoholic or addict, it may be the perception that the nightly glass of wine before supper is dulling his or her intellectual sharpness more than is acceptable; for another, it may be the loss of a job; for another, it may be a jail sentence; for another, serious illness with the threat of death.

I think it may be possible that the limits of "when it is too late" can be stretched when the paradigm of cancer care changes from one of poisoning to one of enhancing health. Each one of us is on a continuum between extreme health and extreme illness. Choosing to use interventions that push one more toward health may well alter the timeline of a cancer, delaying or even averting the "inevitably fatal" outcome.

It is also too late when one thinks it is. Again, several authors have commented on cases where a diagnosis, correct or not, has changed the course of the disease and perhaps even created one where none existed. Sometimes it is "too late" if one is thinking of one's continuing existence as a burden to someone else. Conversely, it is not "too late" as long as life contains a goal to be striven for, a problem to be solved, or as long as it remains possible to appreciate love and beauty.

Yes, life is terminal. I would add that it is terminal in the present body, which eventually does wear out. However, I have had communication from Doc, Kathleen and others from the other side. Doc chose to leave, I think, when he decided that the pain was too great, the difficulty was too great, and that he could no longer be effective in the current situation and in his body. Kathleen chose to leave, I think, when she realized her cancer had metastasized, she didn't want to live on oxygen in what she thought to be a worsening situation after ten years of struggle— and she was possibly at peace that her job on the planet was done.

There's a bit of a paradox (or "pair o' ducks," as Doc would say) here. Sometimes the very act of "winding up one's affairs" is life-enhancing because it removes some of the roadblocks that may have created illness in the first place. It is a sort of feng shui—like removing the mess from the table so that you don't have to go around it three times to find the thing you just put down. And then, when it has really become impossible to sustain life any more, one's affairs are in order and the job is done, and it is possible to go in peace. We used the healing circle to give Wilhelmina the strength to do precisely that.

Resources

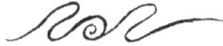

Guided Imagery Tapes/CDs

Belleruth Naparstek
phone: 800-800-8661

Nutrition Consulting

John Cartmell, Clinical nutritionist and massage therapist, Redmond, WA, (phone) 425-883-7444. www.dietadvisor.com. Has nutrition information on cancer and other topics available online. Knows what he is talking about; has been there. Especially knowledgeable about digestion, radiation, leukemia.

Source: John Cartmell; *Townsend Letter*

Treating cancer with Gerson protocol:

The Gerson Institute
PO Box 430
Bonita, CA 91908-0430
Toll-free phone: 1-888-4 GERSON
www.gerson.org
email mail@gerson.org

Treating cancer with Kelley protocol:

Nicholas Gonzalez, MD
36 East 36th Street, Suite 204

New York, NY 10016
(212) 213-3337

Has worked with pancreatic cancer, among others.

Source: *Townsend Letter,* Nov. 2006

His letter immediately follows mine.

One thing that seems interesting about the Kelley protocol is that there are ten different types of diets, therefore making more allowances for individual differences than Gerson does.

Nutritional testing and information:

Health Equations: Takes standard blood test results and analyzes by computer to discover problem areas in nutrition and metabolism. Lynne August, MD will work with your clinician to come up with a protocol for you. I have used this service twice myself and found it amazingly accurate. If your primary goal is to restore health as opposed to killing cancer, this is a great resource! *www.healthequations.com,*800-328-2818. Also articles online on Water and Salt, Cholesterol, Monitoring Hormone Therapies Safely.

www. acucell.com. They have some good articles on vitamins and minerals and their interactions on their website. They also do testing.

Source: John Cartmell

Direct Labs: They do the bloodwork required for the Health Equations Blood Test Evaluation for $97; ask for Comprehensive

Wellness Profile #1. You can order it yourself; your doctor doesn't have to. *www.directlabs.com,* 800-908-0000; for an order form, 800-728-9048. Not available in NY or NJ.

Cancer Testing:

AMAS (Antimalignin Antibody in Serum) Oncolab
36 The Fenway
Boston, MA 02215
phone: 800-922-8378
www.oncolabinc.com.

Blood test particularly useful in early detection and monitoring. Elevated in active immune response; normal after successful treatment or in terminal situation when immune system is exhausted.

Oxygen Therapy:

Cell food, *Lumina* (800) 749-9196,*www.luminahealth.com*

Ed McCabe, *Flood Your Body With Oxygen*

www.oxychargedwater.com. A machine that oxygenates water. I haven't tried it yet, but two of my correspondents have, and they like it.

Source: sooz

Blue-Green Algae and related products:

StemEnhance:
888-783-6832
www.stemenhance.com

Source: sooz

Bio-Algae Concentrates,
www.themagicisbac.com.

Developed by Russian scientist Dr. Michael Kirian, this may well be the best blue-green algae product available at this time

Source: sooz

More information on allopathic and "alternative" treatments:

The Townsend Letter
911 Tyler Street,
Port Townsend
WA 98368-6541
phone: 360-385-6021
fax: 360-385-0699
www. townsendletter.com.

Excellent articles by some of the top names in alternative medicine; one or two issues a year are devoted to cancer. One of the most reliable information sources out there.

Ralph Moss, Ph.D, www.cancerdecisions.com. Writes a regular column in *The Townsend Letter.* Will prepare reports for you on your condition. If you have used his services, please let me know so I can pass the word on. Author of *The Cancer Industry* and *Questioning Chemotherapy*; one of the best-known writers about alternative cancer treatments and about the pitfalls and drawbacks of conventional treatments

The Cancer Control Society, www.cancercontrolsociety.com, sponsors a seminar in Los Angeles once a year, usually over Labor Day Weekend. Following the seminar, they organize a tour of the Tijuana cancer centers, and may also have tours at other times of the year.

Source: *Townsend Letter*

Information on mercury toxicity, dental amalgam, biological dentistry:

DAMS (Dental Amalgam Mercury Solutions, 651-644-4572, www.amalgam.org., is "a non-profit...that educates the public on mercury amalgams and other ways that dentistry may affect health." This organization has a list of books and DVDs available on this subject, maintains a list of dentists practicing biological dentistry, and has staffers available to answer questions.

Sources: Mimi Kuester, Beth Segali

Books and websites:

Maurice Emeka has written two books, *Fear Cancer No More* and *Cancer's Best Medicine*. Following the death of his wife from cancer, he has done his own research. His writing is delightfully simple and straightforward without being simplistic. "Cancer is not a tumor; it's a process," he stated in a recent letter to *Townsend Letter*. I like this kind of thinking. Website: www.cancernomore.com

Guided Imagery and Music: There is more than one type. The one I used was the Helen Bonny Method. E-mail office@ami-bonnymethod.org. Website:www.ami-bonnymethod.org

Joy Indomenico, MT-BC, FAMI
In-Harmony Music Therapy
1049 Main Street, Suite C
West Barnstable, MA 02668
phone 508-280-8618
inharmonymusictherapy.com
joy@inharmonymusictherapy.com.

Individual and small group music therapy with a concentration in the Nordoff and Robbins Improvisational Music Therapy Model; GIM; customized instrumental lessons for exceptional learners and others. My experience with Joy as a GIM practioner was life-changing. Joy is also a skilled and versatile musician and an accomplished teacher who can convey her love of music to students with a wide variety of abilities and learning styles.

Herbs and herbalists:

East Coast:

Jean's Greens
1545 Columbia Turnpike
Castleton, NY 12033
phone: 518-479-0471
www.jeansgreens.com.

Excellent quality herbs, tinctures, teas, salves, reasonable prices, warm and friendly people. Four + One, their version of Essiac, is inexpensive and does the job. Also be sure to check out their one-page reports on various subjects and their books; they also give classes on herbal topics several times a year.

West Coast:

Mountain Rose Herbs
phone: 800-879-3337

All herbs organic or wildcrafted

Source: Linda Strega

Mushrooms and related products:

Fungi Perfecti
phone: 800-780-9126

Source: Linda Strega

Michael Tierra
L.Ac, ND, AHG,
Treating Cancer With Herbs: An Integrative Approach.

Available from Jean's Greens. Michael Tierra is well versed in both Chinese and Western herbs and has an excellent listing of useful herbs and their effects. This looks like a good one. The Chinese system has a lot to offer in terms of support for people with cancer. It addresses the unique characteristics of the individual rather than putting the disease first.

Kate Gilday
Woodland Essence
392 Tea Cup Street
Cold Brook, NY 13324
phone: 315-845-1515
woodland@richnet.com.

Kate is an herbal and flower essence practitioner who uses both Western and Ayurvedic herbs and methods. She is also a NYS Certified Guide and therefore can tell you not only how to prepare your herbs but also where they grow and how to identify and harvest them. She has been working with cancer patients for thirty years. Good information, down to earth, well presented; she teaches at Jean's Greens a couple of times a year. I find her herbalist's perspective on the different families of vegetables unique and very helpful. Her remedies are interesting and fun and you will probably actually do them! She will either teach you how to prepare formulas or prepare them for you.

Susun Weed
PO Box 64
Woodstock, NY 12498
www.susunweed.com
www.ashtreepublishing.com.

Herbalist Susun Weed is the author of four books, *Wise Woman Herbal for the Childbearing Year, Healing Wise, The NEW Menopausal Years,* and *Breast Cancer? Breast Health! The Wise Woman Way.* Her publishing company, Ash Tree Publishing, also publishes the works of Juliette de Bairacli Levy and some other herbalists.

Her descriptions of nettle, chaste tree berries, dandelion, and other common herbs used for women's problems in *The Menopausal Years* (older version) provided an initial model for my coping with my cancer, which had many similarities to menopausal symptoms. I found her Decision Tree extremely valuable in deciding my course of action. She gives lectures and work-shops at her home in Woodstock and at other locations. Her website contains her home and travel schedules, answers to frequently asked questions, and articles.

Rosemary Gladstar
Sage Mountain Retreat Center
PO Box 420
Barre, VT 05649
phone: 802-479-9825
fax 802-476-3722
www. sagemountain.com
e-mail: sagemt@sagemountain.com

Rosemary Gladstar has been a major force in shaping herbalism as it is today. Many well-known herbalists have apprenticed with her at one time or another, and she organizes the International Herb Symposium and the Women's Herb Conference, two important events in the Northeast. Her concern over the possible depletion of herb stocks led to her founding of United Plant Savers, dedicated to the preservation and use of herbs.

Jean Giblette, High Falls Gardens
Box 125
Philmont, NY 12565
www. highfallsgardens.net

High Falls Gardens specializes in growing Chinese herbs in the United States and is part of a consortium of growers doing this work across the country.

Supplements:

Standard Process
1200 West Royal Lee Drive
Palmyra, Wisconsin 53156
customer service: 800-558-8740
home office: 800-848-5061.
www.standardprocess.com

Available through healthcare professionals. Most of their ingredients, with the exception of those of animal origin, are grown on their organic farm. Supplements are derived from whole foods. One of the oldest supplement companies in existence and still one of the most reputable. Founded by Dr. Royal Lee, a dentist, who found that many of his patients' problems stemmed from malnutrition and did much important research that was years ahead of its time. Dr. Lee was therefore vilified by the medical establishment, and the federal government ordered much of his research burned.

I have done well with their products in conjunction with the Health Equations evaluation.

Lymphatics and Circulation:

White Flower Analgesic Balm,

Source: Jarka's Nutrition Center
1618 Grant St.
Bettendorf, IA 52722
phone: 563-359-3157

Chiropractic and Nutritional Support for People with Cancer:

Dr. Jaroslava Odvarko
1618 Grant St.
Bettendorf, IA 52722
phone: 563-359-3157

Protocel
www.protocel.com.
Not to be used in conjunction with Essiac.

Source: Dr. Odvarko

Bodywork/Massage:

Maya Abdominal Massage. For a practitioner in your area, or for self-care classes and information on certification in this modality, *www.arvigomassage.com,* or contact The Arvigo Institute, LLC, 77 West Street, Antrim, NH 03440, (603) 588-2571, at-mam@tds.net. Dr. Rosita Arvigo, a naprapath, studied in Belize for ten years with Mayan shaman Don Elijio Panti. So this proto-col blends naprapathy, which is similar to chiropractic in its focus on the importance of the spine as a modulator of the nervous system and therefore of organ function, and the Mayan traditional style of bodywork and herbalism. Dr. Arvigo's lists of symptoms and causes of uterine malpositioning are an eye-opener—anyone with uterine fibroids, uterine, ovarian or breast cancers, painful or heavy periods, fibrocystic breasts, or any gynecological issues should investigate this material. I find it confirms my hypothesis that there is a connection between uterine distress and diaphragmatic malfunctioning and hiatal hernia. Dr. Arvigo's self-care protocol has been very useful to me in moderating the bleeds.

Four levels of coursework are offered: the Self-Care level is open to anyone. The Professional, Certification, and Certified Teacher courses are open to licensed practitioners who have taken the Self-Care course and the level below.

Tai Chi/Qigong/Medical Qigong:

National Qigong Association NQA,
PO Box 252
Lakeland, MN 55043;
phone: 888-815-1893
www.nqa.org

A good resource for finding a practitioner or teacher near you; they have a membership directory which includes several top names in the field. They give a conference once a year, usually late summer/early fall, in various locations around the country.

Medical Qigong can be a good way of getting in touch with and engaging the energy of your uterus, "quite powerful, not subtle." Recommends a practitioner who trained with Jerry Alan Johnson, OMD, who has written a comprehensive book on Traditional Chinese Medicine.

Source: Susan Richey, L.Ac.

Dandy Blend Herbal Coffee Substitute:

Goosefoot Acres
3283 E. Fairfax Road,

Cleveland, OH 44118,

phone: 800-697-4858

www.dandyblend.com.

Great stuff! Tastes like coffee but has no caffeine and is good for you! Dandelion root is good for liver and kidneys. Also contains extracts of roasted barley, rye, chicory root, and beetroot. Gluten free. Not widely available; ask your health food store to stock it.

Edgar Cayce Material:

Association for Research and Enlightenment

215 67th Street

Virginia Beach, VA. 23451-2061

phone: 757-428-3588

fax: 757-422-4631

www.edgarcayce.org.

Their library is a terrific resource for information on many health and metaphysical topics. A.R.E. Health Center offers massages, colonics and other modalities referred to in the readings. The Lymph Cleanse I use consists of a castor oil pack, acupressure, colonic, and Manual Lymphatic Drainage (the Dr. Vodder method.). They also have a bookstore, 800-723-1112. Membership gives you a discount on Health Center services and A.R.E. Press books. Conferences on many topics throughout the year.

Gladys T. McGarey, MD, a pioneer in the use of Cayce remedies and a founding member of the American Holistic Medical Association, gives seminars on Living Medicine and contacting the Physician Within the patient. The Foundation's efforts also include projects to improve the quality and availability of health care at home and abroad, particularly relating to prenatal care and childbirth. Her humanistic and compassionate perspective is sorely needed at this time!

Dr. Gladys T. McGarey Medical Foundation
4848 E. Cactus Rd.
Scottsdale, AZ 85254
phone: 480-946-4544
www.mcgareyfoundation.org

Cayce Products:

Heritage Store
314 Laskin Road
Virginia Beach, VA 23451.
phone: 757-428-0500
www.caycecures.com

They stock many products recommended in the readings as well as other health foods and supplements. I always stop in the cafe for a sandwich and carrot juice when I'm in Virginia Beach. I also love their bookstore. The Heritage Center also offers massage, chiropractic, osteopathic, and psychic services and classes on various topics..

Catalog orders:

PO Box 444
Virginia Beach, VA
23458-0444,
phone: 800-862-2923

Some of the more common Heritage products, such as castor oil, may be available through your local food coop.

CayceCare Products, *Baar Products*
PO Box 60
Downington, PA 19335,
phone: 800-269-2502 or 610-873-4591
www.baar.com

RESOURCES is a work in progress. I would appreciate your feedback—people, products and services you've used and like, with your comments; also, if I've made any errors, inaccuracies or typos, please let me know! The more input I have, the more inclusive and correct this list will be.

Acknowledgments

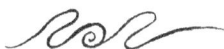

With love and gratitude to the many friends and family who helped me in so many different ways. To the many friends who supported me in my choice not to use conventional medicine and trusted me to do the right thing. To the patients who stayed with me through good and not-so-good times.

It takes an entire village to heal a cancer, and here is mine:

To Sandra Sherrard and Gwenythe Harvey, my inspirations in the early days, who started me thinking about how and whether cancer can be healed by means other than surgery, chemo, or radiation. To Sandra, who was with me the day I received the diagnosis and who first asked me, "Can chiropractic cure cancer?"

In memory of my parents, Helen and William Offenhauser, and of Don Kurtis, Doc Feldman, L. C., and Melba. I learned from all of you.

In memory of Wilhelmina, who worked with me on many healings over the course of the eleven years she was with me;

With love to my sisters, Mimi Kuester, Janet Offenhauser, and Fran Offenhauser, whose spirit of cooperation and dedication made my mother's last days the best they could be, and who supported me in every way when I was sick;

To The Crew, Jean Brower, Teresa Stickle, Shirley Decker, and Jim Humeston, who were always there when I needed them. I could never have built the practice to the level it reached in the busiest days without your constant support in so many ways, large and small. Jean, along with Dr. Fran and Joy, gave me several books at the beginning that helped me shape my strategy for coping with the cancer;

To Toni Van Loan, our "fifth sister," who provided expert real estate advice and practical assistance during the move from the old office to the house in December 2000, and who has always been there when needed;

To Frank Clarke, computer genius and friend;

To Olive Chambers, who cared lovingly for my mother and for me. I remember the many conversations about herbs and about life we had around the kitchen table. We couldn't have done it without you;

To Dr. Lynne August, a true colleague, who has helped me increase my understanding of nutrition;

To Jenny Fairservis, L.Ac., who started me on many of the protocols I still use today, and who reminds me to take care of myself;

To Joy Indomenico, whose Guided Imagery and Music sessions were to become such a vital part of my healing process, who was a staunch friend during the darkest days, and who provided a safe haven for my writing the beginnings of this book;

To Fran Pennix, D.C., my National College and Chicagoland friend, with whom I have shared many adventures, music and folk dancing, and a free exchange of ideas over many years, who first introduced me to the AMAS Test;

To Sharon Kroeger, owner of the unique and invaluable Calsi's General Store, who helped me negotiate the maze of Workers' Comp cases in the early days, who made many healthy meals for me, who is conscientious about stocking the supplements I ask for, and who has created a little center of community around her table;

To Bill Kroeger, grower of beautiful and healthy greens;

To Polly Pitts-Garvin, massage therapist, who worked with me soon after the diagnosis, and helped me begin to see the scope of the work that still remained;

To Dr. Heather Gansel, without whom I would no longer have a practice;

To Barbara Deutsch, M.S.W., who rented office space in the house and made it possible for me to buy it, who joined us for the first healing circle, who offered emotional support during the worst times, and who was always willing to exchange ideas that benefited us both;

To Martha Zimiles, who always had a kind word, a listening ear, and home-grown vegetables;

To Tonia Shoumatoff, companion on the road and cinematographer at the talk I gave in April 2005;

To Karen Triebel, whose Kundalini Yoga class has been a constant source of community for us, and to Vicki Volinski, who does sacred work with the plants and animals. Both of these women took excellent and loving care of Wilhelmina in her last days;

To Dona Ferry who, along with Tonia, organized the first healing circle and generously provided the space for the talk and for our yoga class;

To Susan and Bruce Thompson of Still Point Farm, who sustained me through the Lyme disease and cancer years with beautiful, organically grown vegetables;

To KJ (Katherine Grealish), who provided a gathering place and delicious health food for us for ten years;

To Betty Clegg and the members of the Lombard Reiki share;

To Mary Beth Prosapio, with thanks for that important hypnosis session;

To Mary Stuever, friend and tour guide extraordinaire, who introduced us to Billie Topa Tate;

To Don, Virginia, and Wayne of the Geneva Al-Anon group; to Ramona and others from the Stanfordville Al-Anon group— thank you for giving me the tools to maintain sanity through everything;

To Ray Bayley, D.C., whose lectures on self-care at National College still inform my talks on the subject today;

To Drs. Gregory Cramer and Susan Darby, for that lecture on the skull at National College that was worthy of a round of applause;

To James Winterstein, D.C., president of National University of Health Sciences, who on two occasions has taken time from a busy schedule to write me a personal note, responding to my submissions to the *Alumnus* magazine about the cancer;

To Patrick Nelligan, who helped Judith with computer issues, along with Reverend Dorothy Reinhard, Victoria Reap and Lightning Heart, who welcomed Judith when she was staying with me. Reverend Dorothy is our priestess and herbalist, celebrant of the Wheel of the Year ceremonies that keep us in touch with the seasons, and Victoria and Lightning Heart have a genius for seeing what's needed around the house and finding a way to do it;

To Judith herself. We learned together;

To Rev. Carl Franson, formerly of Sharon United Methodist Church, whose quiet generosity of spirit helped create a welcoming place for us there, and whose automotive repair ministry has benefited Teresa on many occasions;

To the warm and loving people of the Sharon United Methodist Church;

To Linda Strega, whose insightful comments have helped shape this book, and who is always willing to share the wisdom of her experience;

To Rev. Belinda Maund, "Belinda the psychic," who has been accurate on so many occasions, and who predicted this book;

To John Çartmell, nutritionist and massage therapist, who has been generous with his insights into the interplay of nutrition and cancer;

To herbalist Susun Weed, whose book *Menopausal Years* gave me a concept on which to base my treatment of the cancer, which was so very like menopause in its manifestations, and for her wonderful Decision Tree that was so helpful to me in deciding on the order of interventions I chose;

To Holly Applegate, owner of Jean's Greens, whose store is a delight and a treat for the senses, and whose herb classes have helped us learn more and try more things;

To Dr. Gladys McGarey, pioneer on the path to Living Medicine. I hope this book is worthy to be considered a continuation of your work;

To Beth, sooz and Susan, who share their stories and their healing strategies with me and give wonderful support;

To my editor and publisher, Patricia Horan, who believes in the book and keeps asking me to explain one more thing to make it richer and more useful, and who has made it far better than I could have done alone;

To Beth Shaw, our art director, whose inspired choice for the cover captures the theme of this book;

To Sally Reagan for her financial wisdom;

To Jude Streng, our gratitude for first suggesting we investigate Tong Ren healing, and for her artistic eye, skill, and generosity of spirit;

To Stuart Horowitz, for his astute researching;

To Andrei Zimiles, our internet ace;

To the women who have called to ask for guidance and support —thank you for sharing your experience so that we all may learn, and to The Team for their help and encouragement during all stages of this project, and for their brilliant work with the stock market.

Appendix A

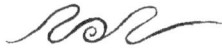

What I Know about Endometrial Cancer

Reprinted with permission from *The Townsend Letter,* November 2006

I originally wrote this piece in April 2005 to use as a handout for the talk I gave at that time and included it as a sidebar to the letter I wrote to *The Townsend Letter* printed in November 2006. Comments in brackets represent clarifications or things I learned subsequently.

1. It can be healed by natural means.

2. Cleaning up the metabolism is of the utmost importance. Otherwise, nothing else will work.

3. Flooding is part of the healing process and should be encouraged, not stopped. It is self-limiting. It can be induced with chaste tree berries or with acupuncture. Sometimes, the body will do it spontaneously. It is responsive to the moods of the body and external events.

4. The healing process is nutritionally expensive. Iron, B
    vitamins, water, minerals, and electrolytes particularly
    need to be replaced. It is possible to compensate for the
    blood loss and reverse anemia. Carotenoids are particu-
    larly helpful. [I was talking about naturally-occurring ca-
    rotenoids here, such as those in juices, not synthetics. Dr.
    Lynne August advised against using iron supplements, as
    cancer cells like iron, and recommended getting addi-
    tional iron from red meat instead. Nettles are also rich in
    iron.]

5. Flooding usually brings emotional upheaval with it,
    pointing out what issues need to be addressed. [Possibly
    exacerbated by caffeine.]

6. It is best to keep bowel and bladder relatively empty to
    minimize pressure on the uterus.

7. The uterus can be adjusted by any one of three methods:
    contacting acupuncture points Ren 4 and Ren 6, the ante-
    rior superior iliac spines [of the pelvis] bilaterally, or the
    symphysis pubis. The latter two change the shape of the
    pelvis, in which it is suspended. This helps with cramping
    and also helps the uterus communicate with the con-
    sciousness.

    [The Maya Abdominal Massage self-care method works
    better than any one of these three; I use elements of all of
    them. Cramping is often accompanied by gas, and adjust-
    ing the lower ribs for hiatal hernia is sometimes even
    more effective than adjusting the uterus itself.]

8. The major problems I had were heat (especially in the
    beginning), sleep disturbances, fatigue, and, of course,

bleeding. Cramping usually occurred when I was eliminating what was probably tumor and was no worse than ordinary menstrual cramping had been. Calcium and magnesium, hot water with cider vinegar and honey, whole milk (especially raw), and crampbark and valerian were particularly helpful for both cramping and sleep. I never had trouble with abdominal pain [other than cramps] or bloating.

[The sleep disturbance can have to do with depletion of the adrenals, and I found that taking a little powdered ashwagandha root at night in yogurt with maple syrup is really helpful! The maple syrup or honey masks the slight bitterness of the ashwagandha. The yogurt helps restore beneficial gut flora as well, and with maple syrup in it, it almost tastes like ice cream.

Another cause of the sleep disturbance was caffeine; at one point I had detoxified to such an extent that a cup of caffeinated tea at lunch would keep me awake at night! Still other causes can be low blood sugar, mineral deficiency, and overstimulation by television or computer late at night.]

9. Anyone with this condition would benefit from Essiac, castor oil packs, and carrot and apple juice, regardless of her ultimate choice of treatment. It has been said that Essiac reduces the chance of spreading cancer during surgery.

10. Cancerous tissue is more viscous and rubbery than ordinary menstrual blood. It ranges in color from bright red to black, according to the state of hydration, and in con

sistency from globs to stringy with beads. Sometimes it is pale bloody mucus, sometimes serous fluid (more of this when the uterus is resting between purges.) The healing process involves tearing down and re-growing of the endometrium.

[The bleeding has gone on for far longer than I ever expected it to. The cancer didn't happen overnight but took years to develop, so it makes sense that this symptom might be slow to resolve. As mentioned above, the bleeding has meant different things at different times. The myometrium was also damaged in the teardown process and therefore also had to be repaired. Periods of prolonged stress have delayed the healing process.]

Appendix B

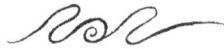

What I Did (Not Necessarily in Order of Importance): A Personal Routine

Reprinted with permission from *The Townsend Letter,* November 2006.

This was the other sidebar included with the original letter. Additions or comments are in brackets.

1. I cut my practice down, cut down number of Workers' Comp patients.

2. I changed my diet, not radically; mostly, I increased greens and improved the quality of food I eat. I eat lots of organic vegetables, especially in summer; salad every day. I find I have much less interest in desserts than I did. I added more animal protein, especially venison, which seems to be what works best. I consume relatively few carbohydrates.

[Venison is harder to get, so I use organically-produced beef from the organic farm nearby. I need this less frequently these days but still more than before I got sick.]

3. Essiac. I'm still doing this twice a day. [I discontinued this in 2007.]

4. Castor oil packs. Daily for about a year, now twice to three times a week.

[I increase these again from time to time, especially if I am having a tendency to athlete's foot or other skin rashes that indicate I am not handlng sugar well, or am feeling irritable and off-center.]

5. Carrot juice [Mostly in the winter now, and not very often; this doesn't feel necessary in summer when raw greens are plentiful.]

6. Seaweed, every day. [Still doing this—2009.]

7. Multiple vitamins, calcium/magnesium, sometimes B complex, sometimes Vitamin C

8. Chinese herbs. [All discontinued in 2007 except Xiao Yao Wan for liver and DBT, a blood tonic, used sporadically]

9. Yoga and Tai Chi, sometimes [Kundalini Yoga class once a week; a couple of poses incorporated into my workout at Curves]

10. Walking just about every day [Getting sloppy. Need to do more.]

11. Acupuncture once a week [Once every 2-3 months— 2009]

12. Dandelion coffee substitute, which tastes like coffee and is a medicinal, good for liver and kidneys. Only caffeine used is caffeinated tea at lunchtime. [I found that even the caffeinated tea at lunchtime was creating a sleep disturbance at night. This took me by surprise. I became more sensitive because of the amount of detoxification I had done.]

13. Lymph Cleanse, every six to ten months [The last one I had was in September 2006. I feel less need to do this regularly, but it's probably time to do it again—2009]

14. I am trying to have more fun and take more time off. [2008 was an exceedingly busy year, and I accomplished more than I have been capable of since before getting sick. Fun and time off have been sacrificed. I need to restore balance in this regard.]

15. Al-Anon, when I get there [not in a LONG time!]

16. Adjusted and communicated with the uterus. She said an assortment of interesting things. [I still do this fairly frequently—2009]

17. I am currently working on organizing the house. Feng shui has a tremendous bearing on my health and my energy. Generally, after a siege of feng shui, the body responds. Cleaning the house is equivalent to flooding, which is equivalent to clearing the emotions.

[2009—This is ongoing. Projects are gradually getting done that were never begun or interrupted due to illness as my energy continues to improve.]

18. Honey, cider vinegar, and Celtic sea salt in hot water at night to help electrolyte balance (always an issue) and aid sleep [2009—Haven't done this recently. Sometimes I use Emergen-C for electrolytes; this worked very well after a short bout of diarrhea recently. Nettle also helps with this.]

19. Guided Imagery and Music, January to June 2003 [Last session July 6, just after the emergency root canal.]

20. Many readings and meditations [ongoing. I find myself getting out of balance if I don't have time to read.]

21. Listening to Mozart, "Heal the Body," almost every night for one year at bedtime. [Don Campbell chose these selections from Mozart for their healing effect. Regardless of how often I hear them, I find them calming and don't get tired of them. I still listen to this sometimes.]

22. Parasite cleanse (black walnut, wormwood, cloves), April 2004

23. Healing prayer, lots of it! [2009—not much lately. I remember to do this mostly in time of crisis. It is also helpful to thank spirit for blessings.]

24. A lot of emotional work

25. I pick and eat herbs from the yard, especially dandelion and violets. I am hoping to add nettle this year. [I started a nettle patch in 2005 which is thriving. Starting in April, I pick enough leaves each day for a pot of tea, eight to twenty-one according to size. There is nothing like the taste of fresh nettle tea—dried nettle, while still full of good nutrients, doesn't approach it! Garlic mustard, a

common weed of the mustard family with the characteristic peppery taste, is good either for spicing up salads or for cooking in the scrambled egg. In 2008, I picked the last garlic mustard in mid-December. I use wild onions and chives as representatives of the onion family. Picking the herbs keeps me conscious of my connection with the earth and the plants that feed me. This is priceless.]

26. Support from friends

27. Chaste tree berries, one month (November-December 2003)

28. Goddess tea for bone and sleep [I'm using straight nettle for this now, since I grow it.]

29. Other herbs from time to time [I added ashwagandha at bedtime about two years ago. I do this fairly frequently, as needed, but not daily.]

30. Herbal Iron for anemia [discontinued 2006 or 2007]

31. I drink lots of water.

32. [Digestive enzymes, occasionally.]

33. [Self-adjustment for hiatal hernia]

About the Author

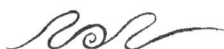

Dr. Nancy Offenhauser is a chiropractor running a unique neighborhood practice in Amenia, NY. A native of New Canaan, Connecticut, she graduated from Smith College and is a 1993 graduate of National College of Chiropractic in Lombard , Illinois, where she also studied acupuncture. Her style of practice has been influenced by the writings of Bernie Siegel, Deepak Chopra, and Norman Cousins, all of whom helped her begin to understand the almost infinite changeability of the body.

Recently she has studied with Lynne August, MD— who has developed a computerized method of analyzing bloodwork based on the work of Emanuel Revici, MD—and with Gladys McGarey, MD, a founding member of the American Holistic Medical Association and a pioneer in the application of the medical intuitive work of Edgar Cayce.

During the last few years, Dr. Offenhauser has been investigating the ways in which the body continually communicates with the consciousness, and is developing theories of personality based upon this work.

This is not the first opportunity Nancy Offenhauser has had to pioneer. She was the first woman stagehand to have a Union card, and worked as a stagehand for many years, on Broadway and off-Broadway, as well as for the ballet and television. A musician who plays five instruments, she has served the theater from the orchestra pit as well.

Dr. Offenhauser's father, William Offenhauser, was also a scientific pioneer, contributing greatly to the development of 16 mm film, stereophonic sound, and television.

Index

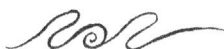

Please visit these websites:

www.healingcancerbook.com
www.healingcancerpeacefully.com
www.theroundhousepress.com

.

www.ingramcontent.com/pod-product-compliance
Lightning Source LLC
Chambersburg PA
CBHW031144270326
41931CB00006B/139